My Liturgy of Easy Walks

Finding the Sacred in Everyday

(and some very strange)

Places

My Liturgy of Easy Walks

Finding the Sacred in Everyday (and some very strange) Places

Copyright © 2022 Marjorie Turner Hollman

ISBN: 978-0-9892043-9-2

1.Non-fiction 2.Memoir 3.Inspiration

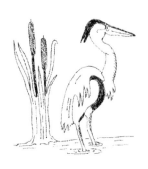

Table of Contents

Introduction

Some books are written quickly. This one has taken almost thirty years to pull together. During this time I've written countless essays reflecting on a life altered by divorce, illness, and healing. The title, *My Liturgy of Easy Walks*, helped form the outline of this book.

"Liturgy" can mean a written order of worship, and can also describe "a way of meeting God." In this context liturgy takes on the widest interpretation of finding God. It has been a guiding principle in choosing each essay that is included here.

Getting outside has been a place of solace, peace, challenge, and joy for me. Easy Walks have become an essential part of my physical and spiritual recovery. Discovering new trails and enjoying the wonder found there is an important part of my family's life.

Among the many stories included here are true tales of how a ball, a bell, and a bicycle, among many other things, became unexpected sources of healing. The loss of both mobility, independence, and continued recovery are challenges I live with every day.

What are Easy Walks? I have learned to describe them as trails that are reasonably level, not too rooty or rocky, with something of interest along the way. *Finding Easy Walks* (the title of my fourth book) and my *Easy Walks* trail guides have allowed me to give back to others. They grew out of my search for places of interest and healing.

Walking, the first chapter, invites you to join me as I get out to enjoy the wonders of creation. *Healing* describes many ways of finding wholeness. *A Child Shall Lead Them* includes both my childhood experiences and stories in which children are the main characters. The title is a biblical reference.

Not by Bread Alone relates stories of preparing and sharing food. These daily occurrences can offer much more than physical sustenance. The title is another biblical reference. *Strength of Family and Friends* emphasizes the importance of friendship and family traditions.

The final chapter, *Lessons Learned*, shares instances of faith, finding grace in small things, overcoming fear, discovering inner strength, and passing on lessons learned to others.

Dates noted along with the title of each essay indicate when it was written. Additional dates in the body of the text give context for when the story occurred.

Walking

Here we focus on both the physical and spiritual act of walking, which can be part of a spiritual practice. As in life, undertaking a journey requires that we take that first step, and can make all the difference.

Many can hike for miles. Others of us struggle to take a few steps. Regardless of how far we can go, or how graceful our movements, taking a walk has the potential to be more than simple exercise.

As an adult I lost the ability to move. My recovery has been slow and difficult. I have fallen (literally) many times along the way. Learning to find and enjoy safe outdoor places while I have continued to regain mobility has been life-giving.

Embracing Seasons of Change—2000

I am keenly aware of seasonal changes, having lived in New England the past forty years. Sap and snow ebb and flow according to seasonal commands that appear erratic at times, yet always push onwards into the next season. There is a knowing that is much larger than any temperature gauge we use for clues about how to dress for the day. The weather reports never tell the whole story.

And so with anniversaries. Birthdays, death days, weddings, divorces, and momentous times mark changes in individual lives, even as the world continues its seasonal rhythms. When I forget to listen, dark times come round and knock me flat. Ignoring, hoping to remain oblivious, doesn't work. There is no escape. I think I am through it. My body knows better. There is no other way but going through.

I would ask for unmitigated joy and celebration. It is denied me. In the midst of what might be a time of celebration, I return to deep mourning for the near loss of my life those years ago. Lingering reminders of earthquake-like changes remain.

My body remembers the sudden sharp shock as a grand mal seizure overtook me, wracking me for ten minutes. Feelings intrude of invasion, loss of control, the effect of planning my own funeral, desperate to insure the well-being of my young children. My sense of bewilderment returns, bringing me back to that time after surgery when I stared at my motionless limbs resting at my side. The fact that

I could feel gave my doctors hope that I might heal from the paralysis. Despite this positive perspective, my only feelings were aching and pain. My healthy limbs cried out for movement, to no avail. That would come later.

Times of exhilaration return despite other memories. Joy tempers the sense of discouragement. A roller coaster of emotions is my constant companion. I should know by now that these low times will come, yet they still catch me unawares.

And then, somehow, a still, small voice says,

Embrace it all.

I really don't want to right now. Thanks, anyway.

Stop fighting. Your body is wiser than you are right now.

If I stop fighting, what will happen?

You'll have to wait and see. It's a story. No one gets to know the end, or even the middle of the story, only the storyteller. Just listen.

I don't want to.

Your body is listening, even if you don't want to. Stay with your body.

It hurts.

I know. Allowing your body to struggle alone hurts even more. Don't leave your body. It is part of you, and needs you very much.

It betrayed me.

No, it has stayed with you, and not abandoned you. It is rich with life, love, energy, excitement, humor, wit, laughter, music, dance, passion, caring, nurturing, compassion, intellect, thoughtfulness, and more you have still not discovered. Don't you want to know what else is waiting in this wondrous gift I have given you?

Not always. Not today. Maybe tomorrow.

Tomorrow may be soon enough.

What if it's not?

You're asking for the next part of the story?

Well, yes.

You will need to listen closely.

How?

You must start by listening to your body. It is a real part of the story. You can't find out the rest if you leave out a huge portion. You will never find out the rest if you leave out the middle. It won't make sense.

Really?

Yes, I promise.

I can't do it alone.

I know. You don't have to.

It feels lonely.

I know.

I hate it.

Hating anything gives more power to what you hate. Loving, embracing, allows it to be what it is.

I can't.

You will when you can.

How do you know?

Because I'm the storyteller, and I know how all stories end.

I thought you said you couldn't tell me how the story was going to end!

Ah, I haven't told you the whole story yet, only enough to give you hope and light, so you are able to keep listening. For what is the storyteller with no listener?

You make me mad sometimes.

Yes.

I just want to know how it will end.

Then the story will be over and it will be time to go home.

That doesn't sound so bad.

There may be some things you might be sorry to have missed.

Why can't you just tell me?

Then it wouldn't be a story.

I hate stories!

Do you?

Well, not really, if I know the storyteller will keep telling me the story.

I will.

You promise?

Yes.

All right. I'm ready.

Oh, good. For once, there was a girl....

Walking in the Rain—1997

Everything else in my life was falling about my ears. It was 1985 and my first marriage was crumbling in front of me. It hurt to stay in the house with so much anger and disappointment. Outside, rain fell in sheets. My two-year old daughter slept. My estranged husband moved about the house making plans that did not include me. My six-year old son bounced on the verge of getting yelled at just because he was six and in a place of terrible upset.

I looked out, turned to my son, and said, "Let's get our coats and boots on," and off we went. We brought along a bright yellow umbrella, which offered a simple shelter to cuddle under, like a portable tent on an adventurous camping trip.

Words came easily as we strode together alongside Silver Lake in the rain. No worrying about getting wet, since we had our boots on, and besides, we could dry out later.

We found streams of water flowing down the street, with sand dams that could be altered to flow in as many directions as a boy wished. We took time to ponder the puddles alongside the lake. Like a small Gulliver in a damp Lilliput, he peered down and decided what should happen here and there, delighted with each result of his careful engineering.

Bits of branches raced and tumbled down the street, headed for the storm drains that emptied out into the lake. Teetering and bobbing, the sticks were finally swept up in waves made by a small boy jumping and splashing near the drain. We went on to look for more log jams and found plenty. The hunt was on.

What a busy hour, for it was surely no more than an hour we spent walking in the rain. It felt like it could go on forever, but it didn't. Not because we were tired, and certainly not because we were bored. We both knew it was time—time to turn for home.

Life was not better there. Yet somehow we were better. We had been in Joy. Home was where we needed to be, sad or not. Anger lurked at every turn as parents were parting, heading very separate ways.

Nothing was fixed by that simple walk in the rain. We never again took a walk that was exactly the same, though we have enjoyed many walks together since that time.

On another day years later, still recovering from the brain surgery that had changed my life, I walked alone alongside Silver Lake in a gentle rain. I listened to the quietness. Gentle plopping sounds of raindrops breaking the water's surface and bird songs echoing against the darkened sky were my companions on this outing. Behind me, footsteps grew closer. My daughter, by then much older than during that remembered walk, came jogging to the end of the lake to meet me. We stopped where the road ended at our neighbor's driveway, made time for her to stretch, then turned, and headed for home.

I walked and she jogged, though I did jog a little, just to show her I was able, despite the changes my body had endured because of lingering irreparable damage to my brain and limbs. Walking was better for me. We spoke of nothing momentous. Sharing companionable joy of being together was more than enough.

As we started up the hill, she broke into a run, turned, and called out, "See you back at the house." Neither wet, nor tired, with nothing pressing that needed to be done, I followed the path home alone.

Lake Life—2010

First published in the Christian Science Monitor *under the title—*
"Lake Life: taking lessons from the local inhabitants." Reprinted with
permission.

I have the heart of a world traveler with the body and temperament of a day-tripper. While I love to hear of others' travels, I have thrived by staying closer to home. By studying one place as it has changed with the seasons and the years, I have learned much about where I live and about myself as well.

Henry David Thoreau noted wryly, "I have traveled a great deal in Concord." Over the years I, like Thoreau, have "traveled a great deal" around Silver Lake, my home of these past many years. This small lake community south of Boston has helped me not only to understand but to make peace with relentless change in my world.

I've observed nesting swans as they hide each year, tucked into the tall grasses at the wilder end of the lake. The newly hatched cygnets' presence is telegraphed by the activity of their parents, heads bobbing in the grasses as they care for their brood.

The Canada geese parade about the lake with their goslings in the spring. The little ones grow fast as their watchful parents guard them and hiss at any who come too close.

With the setting of the summer sun, great blue herons fly to the top of the pines that cover the island in the middle of the lake, settling down as the tree limbs bow under their weight. The geese, giving flying lessons in the fall, provide a front row seat on parenting in the wild, as they insist their young learn to trust their own wings.

I have also watched ducks paddle about the lake with their young, only to count fewer and fewer little ones each morning, as snapping turtles feed on the ducklings. The swans are also often left bereft of their entire parade of young.

In the heat of summer, I have been drawn to the lake many times in search of cool breezes. The coolest places in summer are where the bitterest winds of winter blow.

One February morning I braved the cold, craving the sun and even more the solace of the lake. The swans had been sitting out in the middle of the frozen lake that past week—curiously, in the windiest spot. This day, they looked restless. They shifted and adjusted themselves on the frozen surface.

I left the large birds to their sitting and continued on my way. When I looked again, the two swans had gotten up. Now walking on the ice, their strides telegraphed quite different demeanors. The lead swan strutted, head held high, each step strong and confident. The second swan tucked her head down, wings almost dragging along the cold, hard surface, as if to help maintain her balance. With every step her feet slid.

Suddenly, the first swan began running, full of assurance. The anxious swan ran as well, wings still dragging, head and neck straight out, determined not to be left behind. I could hear feet slapping the ice. Then they were airborne, the sound of their wings echoing across the lake. They lifted up slowly and headed around the island, circling skyward.

We all confront challenges—sometimes with confident grace, other times slipping and sliding. I have always wished to behave gracefully through these times, yet more often find myself slipping and sliding. How fortunate I have been to be surrounded by such wise teachers.

An Easy Walk—2016

Some people think I'm a high-level walker, able to leap tall bushes at a single bound. In reality I clump along as best I can. I take Easy Walks, since I'm not up to tackling more physically demanding trails. I was a strong hiker a long time ago. Since that turning point in my life now many years in the past, I've lived with total paralysis of my right leg that has transformed into partial paralysis. This is not always evident to casual observers. I love to take Easy Walks, yet they really are the only kind of walks I can manage, with support.

The most important support I have is walking partners. My husband and I walk almost every weekend, if we're not out on our tandem bike. During the week, I plan exploratory or simple visits to favorite outdoor places with friends, family, and other interested folks.

Just as when I was first relearning to walk, Silver Lake in Bellingham has continued to be my go-to spot to heal. Our house is near the lake, so it's a short walk to the water, an Easy Walk for me.

One day I kept my eye on a nesting swan and hoped to get a glimpse of her cygnets, which surely had hatched. Alas, when I reached the end of the road that follows the shore of the lake, the swan was "feathering her nest," making things more comfortable, or perhaps simply finding something to do as she sat, and sat, and sat! No little ones were in sight. Dawn or dusk would offer a better chance to spot cygnets paddling behind their mother. Not that day.

Instead of seeing cute baby birds, I was content to watch trees blown about by the gusty winds of spring. Flowers bloomed, bees drank their fill from the blossoms in neighbor's yards, and the oak trees began to shift to a lacy green rather than the bare branches that had stood bare all winter.

I love to explore and find new places to walk, yet as many before me have said, there's no place like home. And lucky for me, home offers an ever-changing landscape each time I venture to the shores of the lake.

Walking in Another's Shoes—2017

I met Liz along a trail as we joined others who had ventured out to help with a trail cleanup. For those who have never participated in these events, they are very social. Yes, we're making the trail cleaner, but if you're not careful, you might make friends who will change your life. Liz is one of those friends—indomitable, determined, clear in what she needs and what she wants, and creative in figuring out how to meet those goals.

Liz is also visually impaired. Blindness is not something she grew up with, so she has had to adapt to this change as an adult. After learning she would lose her sight, she altered the direction of her legal profession and retrained to become a disability and elder-law attorney. As an advocate for the disabled, she has found creative ways to help others with disabilities to become more active. She has also worked to encourage those without overt disabilities to get acquainted with and learn from her visually impaired and otherwise disabled friends.

Her indoor winter walking program encourages people who are visually impaired to be more active. A secondary goal is to introduce sighted individuals to those who are visually impaired, encouraging them to learn from each other. I attended a walking event with Liz and made some discoveries.

My first surprise was that Saint Vincent's Hospital is a great indoor walking space in Worcester, Massachusetts. The trees are real, a waterfall cascades for three stories, and the walkways are broad enough for friends to walk comfortably next to each other. I was told that the gardens would be filled with spring bulbs bursting into flower when the weather grew warm.

After some formalities, we were paired up, sighted guides with visually impaired persons. As my walking partner and I set off, we realized we were going the wrong way: walkers were expected to travel counterclockwise. Surprise number two.

My companion and I found that thought we had come from different situations, we had much in common. We were born in different countries, and our homes are distant from each other. She is blind, while I have difficulty walking. She nodded as I talked about what was hard for me. As we chatted of home and family, we learned that we were more alike than either of us had assumed when we started.

Arm in arm, we negotiated the walkways. I noticed people brushing past us without saying anything, taking no notice of my walking partner's white cane, a universal sign that someone is visually impaired. Occasionally people said, "Excuse me," as they passed us with care. I might not have noticed this before. With her holding my arm and allowing me to be her guide, I felt the difference. It was plain to see how difficult it is for someone with reduced sight to have others pass by, saying nothing. Surprise number three.

Yet another surprise—though it probably shouldn't have been, once I thought about it—I learned that some who have lost their sight as adults resist carrying a white cane that would alert others that they are blind and might be in need of assistance. I understand that sentiment. The problem is, when help is needed, passersby won't understand the need, and may not grasp the situation. My own unreasonable wish is that others could read my mind, giving me space when I need it and coming alongside me to help when necessary. The last time I checked, mind-reading is still a rare talent.

And so I walk, and share my writing. Asking for help is still up to me, or you, if and when you need it. It does get easier with practice. What I also was reminded of by my friends who are visually impaired is that all of us have something to teach others. May we each slow down enough to enjoy the view, be grateful for help offered, and stand ready to offer a hand using the gifts each of us have.

It is not an easy thing to understand how another person feels. "Walking in their shoes," even if it means walking next to them, is a great place to start. You never know what you might learn, so be warned: taking a walk can change your life.

Asking for Help—2017

We arrived on a bright winter day at Birchwold Farm, an open piece of conservation land in Wrentham, Massachusetts. I love to snowshoe, but partial paralysis makes rising from a squatting position impossible for me. I need some help getting strapped in to my snowshoes before I can even get started. Knowing this, my husband Jon bent down and strapped on my snowshoes, tightening the bindings around my winter boots.

The snow was deep so he would needed to break trail for me. We tromped out into the open field. His snowshoes are narrower than my own, so as I followed behind him, each step I took with my snowshoes caught the ridge of crusty snow at the edge of our tracks, threatening my balance. This was not feeling like an Easy Walk.

We headed toward the stream that flowed along the far side of the field. Deer had been through here before us, and their legs had drawn thin lines that sliced through the snow. Exuberant dogs had left their tracks as well as they galloped in random patterns across the drifts. As we entered the woods in search of the water we spied tiny mouse prints that began at the edge of a rock outcropping, then disappeared under the protective snow cover next to a nearby fallen tree branch.

The slope down to the stream felt precarious. I had to focus on each step to avoid taking a tumble. We found the stream almost covered over with overgrown branches and brambles, the wet spots peeking out through the jumble of bushes and snow drifts.

The trees held a heavy snow load from the previous storm, even as more flakes began to fall. As we passed underneath some snow-laden branches, I wanted to take a picture while looking up from underneath the branches. Jon suggested instead that he take a movie of me in that position as he jiggled the tree limbs, sending cold showers of frozen snow over me. I pointed out that this would be a lot more fun if I were the one making the movie and dumping the cold, wet stuff on him. In the end we agreed to leave the snow alone to fall without our help.

And thus we arrived at the last stage of our outing—removing my snowshoes. Once again, he bent down, released the clips on my shoes, and helped me step out of them. He also made sure I got back into the truck without sliding underneath the vehicle. Yes, this happened once. Our marriage does not lack excitement.

It seems such a simple thing—accepting that everyone needs help. And still I chafe.

Silver Lake Ospreys—2011

I never know what I will see on my walks along Silver Lake. Often there is only quiet water, various greens of the oak, pine, and maple trees across the lake on the island, and cloud formations shifting with the wind or changing color at sunset. As the end of the road, the part that many walkers dislike because of the shallowness and weediness of the water, I'm most likely to see the best features of Silver Lake.

This is where the great blue heron likes to hang out and stalk fish with silent stealth. Cormorants may cruise by, climb out of the water and rest on one of the stumps poking out of the water, their wings outstretched to dry in the sunshine. Frogs croak, their calls echoing across the lake, and kingfishers broadcast their recognizable rat-a-tat call as they skim the water's surface, hunting for fish. If I am sharing Silver Lake with a friend, we don't turn around till we've gone as far along the shoreline as we can. The road stops at a neighbor's driveway; beyond his yard lies the feeder stream that creates the lake.

On a walk with my friend, Barbara, the dark shadow of an osprey passed right over our heads. We looked up in time to see this fish hawk settle near the top of an oak right in front of us. It soon took off again, soaring over the water.

We slowed to watch what might happen. Another osprey joined the first, and they both circled the lake, high up, back and forth, hovering over the open water.

"Look! He's going to dive for a fish!" And he did. We stood, mesmerized by this large bird that hit the surface of the lake, seemed to pause for just a moment, then with a great spray of water lifted itself back up out of the water and into the air, his catch dangling from his talons. Once free he then flew straight over the trees and off. The other osprey followed in his wake. They had gone to have lunch. A mallard swimming on the far side of the lake near the island let out a loud "honk!" an "all clear" signal. We laughed.

As we continued our stroll, Barbara marveled at what a wonderful neighborhood I live in, and how much she welcomed sharing the lake with me. I echoed a sentiment I have expressed many times before: "I am very lucky to be here."

Each time I speak these words, the meaning feels deeply layered. Lucky to be alive. Lucky to be alive at Silver Lake. Fortunate to have a beautiful place where I can spend time with friends. Grateful to be able to walk, for it wasn't always so. And once in a while, something beautiful happens, beyond the everyday pleasure of being outside, and I can't help saying "Yeah, I'm really lucky." It's even better when I can experience that wonder with others.

Outward Appearances—2021

Day by day our surroundings seem little changed. The lake is frozen, and snow fills the yards alongside the road, insulating the ground in our neighborhood. Unless fresh-fallen snow alters our views, a monochromatic landscape is our winter scenery.

Trees alongside the water and in the woods behind our house appear unchanged. Bare branches shake in the winter wind that cuts across the expanse of frozen water. Leafless trees wait in quiet throughout the winter, yet hidden in the depths of each of them, secret forces are at work.

In winter deciduous plants (trees and bushes that drop their leaves annually) rest, having shed their leaves the previous fall. Sap settles in roots buried deep in the earth. After each storm, snow-laden branches soon shake off their white coverings to return to their bare starkness. Snow offers needed moisture and a protective covering for the roots that hide underground.

In this time of barrenness we are able to better see the lay of the land, usually hidden by overgrown brush, thickets, and trees. The lack of leaves reveals otherwise hidden stone walls that are often obscured by lush summer greenery. These rocks, stacked on top of one another and tracing lines in all directions, tell us the fields were most likely cultivated for crops. At one time they were open fields with not a tree in sight.

By outward appearances these trees are the same as the year before. Those who know the rhythm of the seasons are preparing to tap certain special trees to steal their sap. Sugar maples are prized— the lifeblood of these trees will be boiled down and concentrated into maple syrup, a treat on many a breakfast table. Warm days in late winter with bright sunshine and cold winter nights stir changes that will soon bring outward signs of spring. Change is afoot deep inside, hidden from view.

Tapping maple trees and hoping to obtain free-flowing sap is an act of faith. Each year we look for the sap to begin flowing upward. Will the trees once again follow nature's pattern and start preparing for spring? Outward appearances notwithstanding, even as snow lays thick on the ground and with no apparent outward sign of spring, change has begun.

Hunting Spring Peepers—2009

I enlisted my young children in the expedition, assembled our flashlights and headed off for Stony Brook Wildlife Sanctuary, our local Mass Audubon property. It was March, 1989, and rather chilly. This is when spring peepers vocalize, looking for mates.

The naturalist greeted us and explained that he would use triangulation to locate these little hard-to-find critters. We were to stand on the boardwalk over the swamp, shining our flashlights where we thought we heard spring peepers. He would get in the water and head to where the path of two lights crossed, hoping to grab a peeper. I was glad to be a spectator rather than the one stepping into cold water in the dark.

Once we were on the boardwalk, we listened. The peepers grew still. They heard us. We waited in silence and before long the peeping resumed. Our job was to focus on one source of peeping, shine our light where it was coming from, and hope that someone else in the group would pick the same critter to focus on.

Stepping into the water, with appropriate groans and squishes, Tom slogged over to where two of our flashlight beams met. He assured us he had done this many times and had always been able to catch some peepers. He dug through the swamp grass—nothing. Not to worry, he assured us. He would find one. We kept up our vigil, aiming our lights, and peering into the swamp, which was dark yet made bright by the light of multiple flashlights.

Tom maintained a cheery patter as he slogged about the edges of the swamp. He was known within the Audubon community as the standup comic of the amphibian and reptile world. This evening I suspect we were having much more fun with our flashlights than he was, as he splashed through the cold water of the swamp chasing elusive peepers.

A man who clearly knew his audience, Tom called it quits when our flashlights began to focus more on the stars than the swamp. He and we had had enough. No peepers. No apologies, just part of the uncertainty and wonder of nature.

On another day, I went on an Audubon outing at a different sanctuary, with different folks, in midsummer. Our group was intent on exploring an upland forest, looking for signs of porcupines. We had just ducked under some hemlocks, searching for whatever we might notice.

I felt clueless, unsure what I was supposed to see. I had never having spotted signs of porcupines, or a porcupine itself. Behind me I heard a woman call out, "Come look!" She had brought with her a little clear plastic collecting box with a magnifying glass built into it. Inside the box was a spring peeper she had scooped with care into the container. Not peeping. Not ready to swim away. Not even in the spring. Just sitting under some hemlocks, minding its own business. Suddenly he was surrounded by a bunch of people who had almost stepped on him.

We all got to see this little wonder enclosed for moment in the collecting box so we could study it. Afterwards we set the tiny peeper down onto the hemlock needles behind where we'd walked. We didn't want to tromp on it by mistake.

Sometimes we have to wait for what we want, or what we think we need. And sometimes the place where it appears is quite unexpected. It's important to step carefully. You never know what might be right underfoot.

Having Eyes to See—2011

"The wall is still here!" the young woman exclaimed as she strode through the grass to the water's edge and poked at the ground with her toe. She called over to her mother, who was inside the car, looking out the window. The two women had stopped to talk to me as I walked along the road by the lake near where I live.

Nearing the end of the road, the car had driven slowly toward me. Stopping, the driver rolled down her window. "We used to live here." She pointed to the house we stood in front of. "We were driving by the neighborhood and my mother said she'd like to see how things had changed."

In a ritual I've developed upon meeting older people who have lived here for many years, I began reciting the names of my beloved elderly neighbors who were now gone, noting anecdotes that brought knowing smiles. Of the few older neighbors who remained, I confirmed that they were still as feisty and friendly as ever, real characters, like any neighborhood seems to have.

The older woman recalled picking blueberries along the lake, yet struggled to orient herself to her erstwhile neighbors and their children and grandchildren. I longed to help. My efforts weren't very successful.

She then motioned to the house, noting that her father had built all the stone walls and the stairs that wound up the hill to the house that sat on a rise overlooking the lake. She wondered if anyone was home. The woman who lived there worked all day, so I said no. She then pointed to the waterfront, indicating that there was once a fence that ran along the edge of the street, as well as a stone wall along the water's edge.

With the mention of the wall, her daughter, clearly curious, turned off the engine and stepped out, leaving the car in the street. She turned to me, laughed, and said, "No one comes down here. We won't be in anyone's way." Some things hadn't changed.

Wandering to the round, stone well, the younger woman poked through the tall weeds growing up around the edges of the structure. "My father built that, too," the older woman told me, nodding in that direction. "When I lived here, we got water from it," she remembered, a wistfulness in her voice. Her daughter, lifting a loose rock, handled it as if thinking about claiming a piece of her former home for a remembrance. Changing her mind, she replaced the stone where she had found it.

Almost at the water's edge, where cattails filled that section of the lake right up to the yard, the young woman paced the length of the yard. Looking back at her mother, she called, "The wall's still here!" I glanced over, with difficulty spotting what looked like stones buried in the grass, foundations of the former wall still embedded in the yard.

What had been invisible to me was bright and clear in their minds. In their eyes, their former home stood unchanged, something I was unable to see.

Visitors—2021

As winter draws to a close I feel reluctant to step out my door. In mid winter I know what to wear, which mittens to pull on, and the right boots to pull on if snow has fallen or if the ground is dry. With spring's approach I must check each day to decide how many layers to pull on, which socks to wear, and which hat to bring along. The seasons are changing again, but I have not kept up.

It is easier to stay inside. Despite my reluctance to adapt, I pause at my kitchen window in case any birds have arrived at the feeder. Ground feeding juncos stray from the feeder and venture near where I stand.

Bluebirds arrive in groups, first one, then a second, and soon five or six perch on the metal pole where our feeders hang. They drop to the ground, hopping across the mostly melted snow. They seem to have no fear of the ice. Their little claw feet grip the icy remnants of a now forgotten snow storm before moving to the bare grassy spots where they hunt for hidden seeds.

Downy woodpeckers visit often. They crave the suet I hang from green wire cages. They and other visitors peck at the fat that provides life-giving food in winter. It will help them stay warm while cold winds blow, even as spring approaches.

When a hairy woodpecker shows up it catches my attention. So much larger than its downy cousins, the hairy woodpeckers appear to be overweight, a suddenly grownup downy. At first glance I wonder if it could be the even larger red-breasted woodpecker, but no, the coloring is not the same. I used to think downy and hairy woodpeckers were indistinguishable, but though their coloring is similar, the size difference is stark. Is it because I have spent time paying attention? Or are these larger hairy woodpeckers, new arrivals in our neighborhood?

Bird visitors at my feeder draw me into the fresh air. I strive to remain still. If I slide our glass doors open, or make a sudden movement, they scatter and the yard returns to stillness. Their presence reminds me that life continues, regardless of how I feel.

Getting outside of ourselves and stepping into another's shoes, even if they are little claw bird feet, can make a difference. Finding hidden seeds can require different skills, discovering alternate ways of seeing the world.

Past and Present—2015

In the past I struggled to survive; on this day, I was on a quest. A quest for what, I was not quite sure. I've lived in one place for more than forty years and have followed the path along the edge of Silver Lake countless times. On my way I've met neighbors, many of whom have become friends. They have grown older, as have I, and many neighbors I knew when I was a young mother have grown old and died. Passing by each house, I think of those who called this neighborhood home, greeted me on my daily outings, and offered a friendly voice during sometimes very difficult times in my life. While they are gone, their presence lingers.

This path has offered a familiar destination for me and my children over decades. Friends have accompanied me, as well as neighbors, family, new acquaintances, and young grandchildren. More often than not, however, these outings have been solitary. This morning's visit to the lake was much the same as other walks, yet I am different.

There was a time when I traced the shores of Silver Lake every day as I slowly recovered after almost dying following brain surgery. It took not just weeks, not just months, but years to regain movement, strength, and hope. These daily outings have helped heal both my body and my spirit.

Near the end of this day's walk, I paused by the dock where my children had learned to swim. To me it will always be Mrs.

Perreault's dock, although the house has changed hands several times since her death. At the end of the dock were neighbors, a dad standing next to his son, who was fishing. The father stood nearby, ready to help if needed. How many times has that dock supported children learning to fish? It has sometimes been a launching pad for energetic kids eager to cool off in summer. I walked down that hill often with my children so we could cool down in the lake on a hot summer's day. Other times we pushed off from the shoreline in canoes or kayaks to explore the lake. On this day I waved at the father and son who were hoping to catch a fish; they waved back then returned to their fishing while I headed home.

There's something unique about this little place I call home. It's not for everyone. You probably have a place you're thinking of right now that's home for you and quite different from mine, and that's as it should be. It brings to mind a story my mother loved to tell about her beloved grandfather. Mom would smile and recall, "He'd say, 'It's a good thing everyone isn't the same, or they'd all want to be married to my wife!'" Then Mom would laugh and say, "And she wasn't very nice, so it was even sweeter that he always said that."

Home means something different for each of us, even as we feel in common that attraction, the need for the familiar, the known, the place we belong. Most of us have mixed feelings about home. It's complicated. And so we walk, hoping to return to a place that is our own.

Sounds of Silence—2020

We were tromping through the drifts on a short walk in new fallen snow when I spotted the tracks. Ha! These were our own footprints— we were retracing our steps, headed back home. We had ventured to an old trolley line rail bed that still stands in the woods near our house. The dirt road cuts a straight line through the trees; the path we took did not. Despite the straightness of the trail we still created a wobbly line as we walked.

I smiled. No, we people do not stick to the lines set out before us. There was much to see on this day after a snowstorm, and our zigzagging path told the story of the distractions I found along the way.

Multiple witch hazel shrubs were weighted down by the snow, their fall blossoms of a few weeks before now frozen in place as winter set in. The stream that had been bone dry all summer was now filled, almost overflowing its banks as it tumbled through the woodland. We spotted another set of tracks made by someone else's snowshoes. We later confirmed they belonged to our neighbor, who had gotten out earlier than we had.

The going was more difficult to navigate through than when we walked through the drifts in our yard. Could the difference in snow depths be a matter of how the wind blew? Our house is perched at the top of a sinuous hill, an esker (a long winding ridge of gravel), the remains of a long-ago glacier that covered this land thousands of years ago. The trolley line path is down below us.

The wetlands between our house and the trolley bed are filled in the spring with an orchestra of spring peepers (the high notes) and wood frogs (the bass notes). In this time of new-fallen snow, the loudest sound as we walked was silence. Road noise was muffled. The still air held the cold. The tumbling of the stream over rocks created an oh, so sweet, pianissimo symphony of water cascading down small changes in elevation as it made its way to the Peters River, and eventually to the Blackstone River, miles south of us.

Winter had begun in earnest. In fits and starts, the change of seasons would take hold. Rain would soon wash snow into the streams, filling them to the brim. More flurries might arrive, or not. As always, we wait and wonder.

Winter Day's Reflection—2017

I often get the feeling I'm crossing into another place and time when I stride through the woods behind my house. We live within sight of Silver Lake, which at one time was the local hot spot for entertainment of all kinds. At the beach, a carousel spun wooden horses around and around in endless circles, and a dance hall offered Big Band tunes in the 1940s. A roller skating rink drew children far and near to the shores of the lake. At one time performing horses dove into the lake from great heights. An older neighbor showed me where the horses supposedly dove from a perch on the island in the middle of the lake.

Life is much quieter here these days and quieter still the day after winter's storm. We headed back to the woods behind the lake to look for animal prints. Signs of wild turkeys were easy to spot. Deer tracks sliced a long, mostly straight line from one wooded section to another. Coyote tracks led in the same direction we were headed, traversing the same paths we take that lead the sand pits.

Long ago the sand-filled landscape was covered with low bush blueberries. Children paid the landowner fifty cents a day for access to the blueberry fields. A neighbor who had grown up within walking distance of the lake told me stories about picking berries there, then walking five miles to the next town to sell his harvest to the local bakery. Both that neighbor and the blueberries are now gone. Forty years after having been mined for its sand and gravel for construction purposes, the land is now recovering, white pines growing in from the edges of the sand hills. The fields of blueberries have not returned.

It is the rail bed that always stops me. One hundred years ago, we had public transportation that came directly to Silver Lake. By trolley, one could travel to Woonsocket, to Franklin, or Milford, all destinations I must drive to these days. Cars were neither common nor necessary. How very different from the suburbia we live in today.

The steel tracks are long gone, but the raised bed the trolleys traveled along remains, a vestige of the efforts earlier generations made to connect communities through public transportation. These days many are putting efforts into creating community rail trails, with the focus on creating infrastructure for non-motorized transit for recreation, and, one hopes, for transportation as well. Mile by mile, these trails are being constructed, often on the bones of old rail beds, managed by town, state, and non-profit groups seeking to connect communities and to encourage us to be more active.

And so we walk, following animal tracks, traipsing through history, as the streams make their way through the snow to the sea.

Healing

After being injured or experiencing an illness, our normal expectation is that we will be restored to our former level of functioning. Some injuries or illnesses, however, do not allow us to return to life as we'd known it. Does this mean that healing is impossible for the unlucky?

Perhaps we need to search for a different perspective on what wholeness is. Altering our expectations, understanding, and acceptance of what constitutes healing can be in and of itself an important step in creating a new life, and discovering ways of making peace with whatever place we find ourselves in.

Healing

A Fancy Cane—2021

A version of my essay was published on the website, "The Mighty— Making Health about People."

When I returned home from the hospital after brain surgery in 1993, I did a great deal of sitting. Getting across a room was an effort; reaching the other end of the house to use the bathroom was a major undertaking. I spent a lot of time observing my healthy, active children and visiting with neighbors from my cushioned rocker in our living room.

By my side, ready at a minute's notice, was the cane I had brought home from the hospital. Ugly stainless steel, four little feet at its base to provide better balance, this cane remained standing even when I could not.

I always knew where I left it. Waving like a buoy in the ocean, it was a constant reminder of what I had lost.

The little hill where I live has four houses at the top of it. The street dead-ends right at the edge of my yard. Years ago, when my children were growing up, the four houses provided the neighborhood with ten or eleven children, depending on who wanted to be counted as children. The end of the street has about two hundred feet of relatively level, quiet road where children could play and have games of football or basketball. My house stands four feet back from the street, and our dining room and living room offered a front-row seat on the "Silver Lake 500" oval race track. The bike riding in the street in those years was almost constant. Dinner was often a neighborhood affair as racers streamed past our window calling out greetings and checking to see when my children could come out to play.

As I watched the bicycle races in front of our house, I noticed that my rather nondescript cane had a rubber handle that looked quite similar to a bicycle handlebar, complete with the little hole at the end of the handle. It was as though it was waiting for streamers, just like those adorning several bikes passing right by my window.

I grew jealous. I wanted to play, too. My shiny silver cane waved at me as it stood upright in my living room, mocking my longings. It could stand alone unsupported, while I needed its help for my every step.

I looked at the hole in the handle, and then at the bikes weaving through the outdoor games in the street, streamers flying from many of their handlebars, and said to myself, *I need some streamers, too.* I had no sooner voiced my wish than the hunt was on. I was humbled by the determination that my parents, who were staying with me that first summer as I began to heal, and my siblings, who were all relatively local, put into this quest. They had some close calls. One shop had just sold out of bike streamers thanks to a mom planning a birthday party for twenty-six. Other stores were out of stock. My sister, Mary Glen, finally had success when she ventured into a party store, where she found iridescent curlicue streamers. She grabbed them and headed for my house.

With what triumph those streamers were presented to me and installed into the handle of my cane. Cinderella had become a princess! Afterwards, everywhere I went, children wanted to stroke the streamers, and, I was delighted—the focus had stopped being on me and why I was having difficulty walking and became all about my decorated cane. With time the curly streamers lost their bounce and grew scraggly. They endured many tugs from curious little ones. Despite their appearance, they maintained their attraction.

It felt silly to imagine my streamers flying in the wind like the children in my neighborhood who sailed past our house on their bikes. Yet I allowed myself to dream. Little did I know then that one day I would meet the man who would come to understand the longings of my heart and would find us a tandem bicycle I could ride on with him.

My wish, a pipe dream as I struggled along with my cane with curlicue streamers, was fulfilled in a manner I never imagined. Each time we climb onto our adaptive tandem bicycle on local and less local rail trails and begin pedaling, I am reminded of this desire, and feel grateful to have seen it become a reality.

Basketball Miracle—1998

It was summer, and I was able to cross a room only when aided by a cane. I had survived brain surgery that spring of 1993 and was angry with the situation I now found myself in. Unable as a single parent to work to support myself and my children and in pain, I felt very uncertain about the future. My body had betrayed me. What I had perceived as solid ground had proved to be an unstable earthquake zone.

As I sat in my rocking chair, I heard the "thump, thump" of basketballs outside my window. The basketball hoop had been a gift to my children, erected by neighbors from funds collected when these same neighbors heard I had fallen ill. The metal circle mounted on a backboard at the top of a tall wooden pole had become a meeting place for children and adults alike, but I sat in my chair indoors, unable to take part in the fun.

A physical therapist came to help me for a few visits shortly after I returned home from the hospital, and I told her of my wish to play some basketball. Being the kind and wise woman she was, she jumped right up and said, "Let's go." Just like that? It's one thing to sit in a chair and wish. It's another thing entirely to have someone say, "Let's try, and I'll help."

She was not someone who took "no" for an answer, and we soon stood in the street in front of the basketball hoop. My hands clutching the ball, I felt frozen with fear. She offered to move my cane to the side, and promised she would hold onto me by my belt.

Dropping the ball felt terrifying. I tottered off-balance. "I've got you," she promised. I let go and the ball bounced right back to me. After another drop and bounce, I moved as the ball bounced almost out of reach. I took a step toward the ball to catch it. Again and again I shifted, the ball was there, and I adjusted my stance to keep up with it.

Just as I had let my own children go as they learned to balance on a two-wheeled bike, my therapist released her hold on me, and it was all right. Strange as it might sound, the support of the ball bouncing up to meet my hands with each step I took helped keep me upright. I hadn't realized that I was balancing on my own until I looked back and saw this wonderful woman standing a distance away from me, hands on her hips and a huge smile on her face. While I still couldn't cross a room without my cane, for a time I was able to stroll in the street, a bouncing basketball my only support.

I finally put the ball down, and using my cane headed back inside. The euphoria remained. We laughed, imagining bringing a basketball along on outings instead of my cane. We giggled at the thought of my bouncing the ball through the grocery store aisles, standing in front of the vegetables as I dribbled the ball.

I did not make huge strides on the basketball court, nor did I work to polish my dribbling technique. Regardless, this "basketball moment" has remained a touchstone, a moment of magic and transformation. I was given a glimpse into a future that held hope of more healing to come. Despite my resistance, my heart began to open to the joy, the necessity, of change.

Have I come to embrace novelty and new circumstances? Not really. However, when healing does occur, I'm often reminded of a time when I could not walk, and yet, with the support and encouragement of a wise and wonderful woman—and something as unlikely as a bouncing basketball—I took my first steps alone.

Letting Go—1999

Well-intentioned people offer varied strategies intended to short-circuit the difficult process of "letting go," whether it be of worries, pain, hurt, relationships, the past in general, or even prolonged grieving. The list of life challenges is endless, and suggestions for how to cope are endless too, yet have been useless in my own experience. I have learned that letting go is something that happens on its own time schedule, not because of trying harder.

There was a time when I watched in amazement as my right side began the process of learning how to function again, after being deprived of movement as a side effect of life-saving brain surgery. At first, my fingers began wiggling just slightly, nothing that I could control, and not to hold anything of weight. After a few days I was offered plastic drinking straws to grasp. Waving them in the air, I greeted my visitors with the news: "Hey look, I'm lifting straws!" as though I was in a weight-lifting competition. I took any ability to move as a win.

After a few weeks, I was able to clasp my fingers into a fist with some relative strength. Unclasping was difficult and laborious. The holding on came first, the letting go much later. Each instance of healing felt euphoric, even as the big picture of how I could manage my life remained a great unknown. I took every positive development as it came, rejoicing when I could. I still had plenty to be concerned about.

Six weeks after my surgery, I was traveling around the halls of the rehabilitation hospital where I was staying in the early days of my recovery. I sailed along the hall in a wheelchair, using my left leg since my right leg was still paralyzed. I used my left hand to turn the wheel of the chair. A staff person at the hospital chastised me, insisting I should be using both hands to push, not favoring my weaker hand.

I did not bother to respond. Her words took me back to a time when I sat in front of my parents' television set on a Saturday morning, watching cartoons with my siblings. A cartoon character grabbed a spinning wheel and suddenly his hand stretched like a rubber band as the wheel spun round and round. I pictured my hand, which only knew how to grasp strongly, taking hold of the spinning wheel rim as my wheelchair rolled along at a good. As in the cartoon, I watched in horror, in my imagination, as my arm stretched, rubber-like, all the way to the bottom of the wheel.

I knew better than to listen to the misguided scolding of someone who had no idea of my abilities. I shook my head in wonder at such foolishness and continued on my way. My reflexes were not yet able function, allowing my hand to release itself from the wheel in time to avoid injury.

This image of my arm turning to rubber and stretching out of shape provided me with a tangible picture, an understanding of why "letting go" might be so difficult for some of us. Perhaps, like me, there has not been enough time for holding on, for strengthening that part of us that must hold on tightly before we can move on to letting go. To insist that one "should" let go when our muscles, physical or emotional, are not ready can cause more harm than the holding on was doing.

When we find the strength, the letting go will happen. Not because of a conscious decision, or from being shamed into taking this step, or for any other reason than that we have held on enough, tightly enough, strongly enough, long enough. Only then will letting go be possible. Not only possible, it will be exactly the right step to take. It will be time.

Tidal Waves—1999

Sometimes my life feels as if I were living on a tropical island, with an adequate shelter and swaying palm trees. Yet this island rests upon an unstable fault line. Most often the waves lap against the shores of my island as soft breezes blow. Without warning the earth shifts, and the ensuing tidal wave wipes out my haven, washing away most recognizable signs of life. When the water recedes to its former level much looks the same, yet my structure is gone, as are the trees. Bits of "stuff" remain on the beaches. As I pick up pieces of debris, the peaceful scene belies the havoc that was wreaked a short time before. I search, hoping to find something I know, wondering if anything will ever feel "normal" again. Perhaps "normal" life will return, but just under the surface the potential for disruption lies in wait.

This is what living with seizures is like in my own life. I sense the fault line that lurks just below the surface. I manage seizure control with medication and lifestyle. Sometimes these strategies let me down. Sudden pain from injury, stomach upset, or life's anxieties may trigger another seizure. I look "normal," whatever that is, so I fool others. For the most part I fool myself.

After a seizure occurs, at first I have no tolerance for anyone. I need to be very quiet, alone, dark and hidden from everything. I can tolerate one person able to stay quiet. They must be willing to do a lot of giving, since I have nothing to give back. Unexpected noise will push me over the edge and invite another tidal wave to wash over me.

At this time all my mothering instincts desert me. When more than one person enters my space, I flee. Whether I'm stirring soup, setting the table, or in a conversation, if my body says flee, I have no resistance.

In time my body will heal, but scars remain. For the most part mine do not show. Inner changes have worn grooves in my soul that I not only acknowledge but am beginning to embrace. I find the pieces that were once a part of me, pick them up, and begin putting them back together. The shelter I build anew can never be the same. I hope the surrounding seas will remain calm, but life itself is not always peaceful. The unexpected is part of our existence, welcome or not. Embracing change can take a lifetime to learn.

Shining Oaks—2000

The year had been a season of loss. My mom had recently died. A few months later, Chris, my neighborhood partner in so many silly adventures and quiet cups of tea, died of cancer just weeks after receiving her diagnosis. I am the first to remind others that death is a part of life, and yet and yet … sometimes it feels too hard. Sitting with these feelings, I looked out my window and caught sight of the oak trees that surround my home.

The bright sun shone through the oaks, early fall light glowing through bronzed leaves that clung to their branches. I really like oaks. They don't get the star billing that is bestowed on maples and other deciduous trees in New England. No fiery reds or blazing yellows. Their reputation for fall color is all about boring browns, dull, not so impressive. As I looked out my window and across Silver Lake, the oaks displayed their own shining glory. Their flashier cousins had finished their show. It was the oaks' turn.

I was reminded of how much I love the fall, the changes of the season warning of darker, colder months to come. Time was approaching for making soup again, drawing on my comfortable sweaters, and pulling out my lap robe, getting ready for quiet reading times.

I have a lot of mixed feelings about change. I am often resistant to altering my physical surroundings, yet hunger for what the change of seasons brings. These positive aspects of change have spanned different experiences such as evidences of healing and encounters with joy in nature.

By drinking in the sight of my shining oak trees that glow only in the morning sun before they grow truly dull brown with the coming of winter, I take courage. Some of these tenacious oak leaves will hold on through the bitterest cold and strongest winds until new life from budding young leaves push the old leaves out of the way, welcoming the coming warmth of spring. This same promise has given me hope as I have waited for healing that might or might not happen.

Chronic Friends—1999

Throughout the early years of my recovery, my path felt less than smooth, my future unclear. I have been blessed with a number of what I call "friends of the heart," who have remained close, regardless of distance and life events that have sometimes kept us physically apart.

A number of my friends and I have chronic conditions, rather varied in their symptoms yet similar in how these conditions impact our everyday lives. We often feel an otherness that sets us apart. Most of us were already friends before we acquired our chronic conditions. We have the advantage of sharing many interests, and we feel a strong sense of "you know what I'm trying to say" when we talk. Conversations often take place over the phone. Our fellowship is widespread and time for personal visits is difficult to arrange in lives stressed by getting through daily life.

Our dark humor, the ability to laugh at difficult situations we find ourselves in, has become a strong tie that binds us. Our laughter is based on a mutual understanding of the absurdities of life and its tenuousness. The joy I feel after a phone call with one of my "chronic friends" is deep and heartfelt.

We are less wary of complaining to one another than with most others, knowing that whining and complaining wears on people's patience. When someone says to me, "Why complain? It never does any good," I often say "I always feel better when I complain." This response often provokes laughter, which is my intent.

I choose my complainees carefully, knowing that not everyone is interested or able to listen to details of what at times can seem intractable and unbearable. Even in the midst of what may seem like impossible circumstances, life go on, and can even offer some amusement along the way.

Do we rejoice in our tribulations? No. Each small triumph, accomplishment, positive happening, or improvement is greeted with joy. We strive to show a willingness to commiserate when life feels hard, and an eagerness to rejoice when something good happens, whatever that good thing is.

Must you have a chronic condition to join this club? No, since in the big scheme of things, life itself is filled with uncertainty and adventures that none of us, being able to look into the future, would greet with open arms. Membership requires an ability to listen well, laugh, and see that we're in this boat together. The time we've been given in this world is short.

Anyone can become a member. It's your choice. Life is chronic, and temporary, a paradox that should keep us laughing until we encounter something else to cry about. When tears are called for, they're allowed to flow. So join the club. You'll find some good company.

Learning to Skip—2001

Ellen was over for a visit, and I told her I might be able to skip again. It was 1995, two years after the surgery that dramatically altered my life. I could sense that changes were happening in my body, but skipping alone felt very scary. Some hand-holding was in order; would she help me? With a smile, she said, "Yes."

Self-consciousness is a life-long affliction for me. I didn't want anyone to see me fail, so we headed down my street and off toward the old trolley rail bed that is now a dirt road leading into the woods. From my house on top of the hill, the path is not visible.

Once we reached the woodland trail in relative privacy, I got up my courage and said, "Let's try it." I lay down my cane, took her elbow, and off we went. I really could skip!

The ability to skip is used as a kindergarten-readiness test. Succeeding in this endeavor, I had passed an important milestone in healing. The sensation of skipping was euphoric. We continued skipping, arm in arm down the dirt road, which might have been made of yellow bricks. After we stopped to catch (my) breath, we walked, then I tried skipping again and achieved the same result—success! I did not, however, factor into the equation an important point.

Not long afterwards, I visited to my brother and his family. I wanted to show them the new healing that had taken place, and tried to skip in their kitchen. By myself. And nearly caused some breakage. We were all stunned.

My mistake was that I hadn't asked anyone to hold my hand. Though I could skip on the arm of my friend, attempting it alone was another matter. I had thought that if I had healed, it would be a complete healing. This was not so. As with so much of my life, I'm able to accomplish many things with support. Undertaking the same task is not only foolhardy, it is inadvisable.

Sometimes I hate that. Other times I see how rich my life has become. It is filled with people I need who seek out my company, not out of pity, but because we enjoy doing things together.

The isolation of independence, of driving as far as I might wish, or running ragged in the frantic pace that seems to be modern American life are not options for me. I learned that some envy my network of support. In time I grew to understand that this was not true envy. Others expressed a longing for the connectedness I had been forced to develop out of need.

This came about as I learned to ask for assistance. I was in the position of having overwhelming needs that showed no sign of going away. I always hated asking for help.

I was unable to drive for seven years after my brain surgery because recurrent seizures prevented me from safely getting behind the wheel of a car. I live three miles from the nearest store and my family all live at least an hour away. Transportation to doctor's appointments, food shopping, and other errands were weekly tasks I was unable to do alone. Neighbors, long-time friends, new friends, and people from church all offered their time.

In those years our area had no public transportation available except for medical appointments scheduled well in advance. The situation has greatly improved. Senior centers have vans to take area resident shopping and to medical appointments. This was way in the future. In the 1990s I was on my own.

My learned to "cast a wide net" as I called it, in asking for help. I telephoned those I thought might be able to meet whatever need had come up, but I always began with "You must say 'no' if this is not a good time, so I can feel like it's ok to ask again in the future." I then told them when and where I needed to go. We had no email at the time, but I had a working phone, and thankfully my voice had not been affected. I thought often about how much more difficult it would have been if I had lost my voice.

Over the years I developed a network of helpers I could depend on. I worked hard not to lean on any one too much, and always prefaced my request with the same, "Tell me if this is not workable for you." Some of those I called were acquaintances who became close friends I still cherish.

Once I began to drive again, with my seizures under control, the change in my daily routine was profound. I saw how easy it can be to become isolated and alone in American society. Years of being unable to drive had forced me to learn to ask for help, and taught me that many like being able to help when they feel respected and not taken advantage of. My altered life fostered strong friendships. These relationships helped me find ways to give back when I was able. My needs had become a tool for establishing bonds that have become mutual. Even when I felt I had nothing to give, others saw me differently and welcomed me into their lives.

When asked if I wished I could go back to my way of life before I got sick, I answered without hesitation, "No!" Further reflection helped clarify that I had no desire to go back to the life I'd lived before, which was filled with frenetic pushing, hurrying, exhaustion, and loneliness. I can't go back. Then again, I don't pray for that kind of miracle, either.

There are many different kinds and levels of healing. That feels pretty exciting. Almost enough to make me want to skip—with a friend.

Stilt Walking—1998

My father built a pair of stilts for us when I was a child, wooden two-by-fours with a triangular wedge for a footrest, which lifted us about a foot or so off the ground. I don't know where he got the idea but they were a great toy. Mounting them, so to speak, took time to learn. My siblings and I, along with other kids in the neighborhood, took turns holding the stilts for one another until we were ready to take our first tentative steps unassisted.

Walking on stilts required coordinating our arms and feet, and lifting each stilt in turn while keeping our feet pressed onto the wedge-shaped foot rests. The stilts were not too far off the ground, helping us avoid serious injury since we often pitched forward, crashing in a heap on the ground, arms, legs, and stilts all tangled, though soon sorted out. Before long, I learned to get myself up unassisted and marched with confidence all over our yard, down the street, along the sidewalk in front of our house, and all the way around the block.

The most treacherous was muddy ground. The posts tended to sink, bogging me down and dumping me off the stilts. Errant children running into my path could throw me off. I flew off in a tumbled heap more than once.

Momentum was most difficult to maintain when moving very fast or too slow. Too quick and I soon pitched over. The opposite was like trying to pedal a bike, the slower the pace, the bigger the risk of tipping over. Gravity is almost impossible to counter when moving at a turtle's speed.

My childhood stilt walking days often came to mind as I learned again to walk. I often felt as precarious as when I navigated my childhood neighborhood on stilts.

As when using stilts as a child, I found, within this changed body, that slow walking was quite difficult. Sustained momentum was essential to remaining upright. When I was pushed to take a class in mindfulness meditation (doctors initially misdiagnosed my seizures as depression and urged me to take the class), we were urged to stop rushing, as a form of meditation. I fumed inside. I was already walking mindfully, aware of each step I took. Decreasing my pace put me off balance and put me in danger of falling. The lessons I learned from the class were probably not what the instructors had intended.

I envied the one-year-old child next door, who, when she grew tired of walking, and whose gait looked remarkably similar to my own, would plop down and continue crawling to where she wanted to go. My adult sensibilities forbade me from resorting to such a logical way of propelling myself. Instead, first with a walker, then with a cane, later with sheer determination, I walked upright, more or less, with a great sense of precariousness and heightened awareness of each step taken.

I wasn't conscious of how precarious my stride was until I read a book by neurologist Oliver Sacks, in which he described how those who cope with neurological deficits do all sorts of compensating to achieve what "normal" people do with little or no thought or effort. Pondering how challenging each walking step was for me, and how I was catching myself with each step taken, I realized my center of balance, unlike most, rested not in my hips, but was down around my knees. It felt very much like I was walking on stilts.

While intrigued by this insight, I felt very frustrated. To others, my gait showed a slight limp. In contrast to how others perceived me, I felt like I was balancing on wobbly wooden posts that threatened to toss me through the air with little or no warning. I grew angry thinking about the energy required for me to move.

A few weeks after this insight, I clunked my way to the kitchen sink and heard a voice inside my head say, "You have your balance back." Right behind this voice I heard another say, "You think you have your balance back." Then a third, "You hope you have your balance back."

I believe in God. I pray, and feel my prayers are heard, but I am not in the habit of hearing voices. All this was very odd to me, so I retreated to my rocking chair to let things sort themselves out.

When I had to stand up again, my center of balance had shifted to my hips. It felt as if I were floating down the hallway of my house. When I woke the next morning, I wondered if the shift in my balance was my imagination. No, the change was real.

I took a walk along the lake and felt so light; it was as if my feet had not touched the ground the entire way. Such lightness, such (comparative) ease. No more walking on stilts.

When I meet those who think that trying harder is the best way to achieve a goal, I tell them this story. Yes, trying harder did help me to master walking on stilts. As a child I could always get myself back down from the stilts. To be allowed to come back down as an adult and walk again nearly as others do was not a result of my trying harder. Before this, I walked as if on stilts, with whatever balance I had. I refused to retreat to my rocking chair and ventured out, even when the stilt walking sensation felt frightening. Then one day, something changed.

I still don't know the reasons nor do I believe that physical wholeness is the only valid goal of healing. I used to walk on stilts as a child and it was great fun. Later, when I had no choice about getting down from my "stilts," it was not nearly as much fun, yet I did it. For that, I'm grateful, since it seems I was given very early training for stilt-walking. When needed, the training had not been forgotten. Now I am able to leave my stilts at home, although tripping is still an ever-present risk. That, however, is another story.

Marjorie Dances—2002

I loved to dance, but lost the ability to move in 1993. After six months, I was able to return to contra dancing, supported by my local dance community. These supportive dancers took great care in keeping me safe as I danced. I leaned on them a lot through the course of each dance, depending on them to provide the balance I lacked, and to walk me back to my seat after each dance. In those early days, I was able to dance, yet could not walk across the dance floor unsupported. Dancing and dancing gracefully are not the same. Walking and walking gracefully are different too.

Friends gave me rides to our local monthly dances. An unexpected gift that came from my showing up became "the Marjorie Dances." And yes, there's a story.

In contra dancing, one person dances in tandem with a partner or a neighbor, often holding hands through portions of the dance, and less often unsupported. It is akin to square dancing, but in long pairs of lines, rather than in squares.

Feeling supported by understanding dancers allowed me to move better in my post-surgery life. Along with the highs of pleasure at the freedom of movement I enjoyed during these dances were the lows when I was reminded of how difficult it could be for me to move at all.

Some contra dancing movements require pivoting in place, often a full rotation. This doesn't work for me. A "hay for four," involves weaving unsupported in and out around the other three people in a group of four. The pounding my right foot takes as I pivot back and forth increases my pain and removes the fun of dancing. My response has been to adapt or decline to do them at all.

One of my dance friends, Bob, had been the recipient of a number of my grumps about the difficulty I had with some of certain dance moves. He is a wonderful dancer, very responsive, and has a great sense of humor. After one challenging (to me) dance he promised, "Someday I will write a dance for you that has only things in it that you like."

I heard nothing more about his promise. Every now and then there would be something in a dance that would irritate me, and I'd say, "None of those in my dance!" He'd nod his head, and then smile. He was taking it all in.

Bob has become a skilled dance caller-teacher, and has called often at our local contra dances. One Saturday night when he was calling at our local dance in Medway, Massachusetts, he pulled me aside and said, "Make sure you're dancing with someone you really enjoy for this next dance." This was before I had met my future husband—at a contra dance! I was slightly puzzled, yet trusted Bob's intention and took the hint. I found a friend to dance with me.

Bob began teaching the next dance, and walked us through each portion, one section at a time. When he felt comfortable that we understood how the dance went, he explained that he had written the dance for me, and had called it "Fun Dance for Marjorie." He hoped that I would, indeed, have fun dancing. He suggested that the other dancers might check with me to see if I was having fun as I progressed up or down the line of dancers, and the music began.

Contra dancing, by its structure, progresses each pair of dancers and up or down the hall, which requires dancing with practically every person in turn who has come to the dance. As I went down the line, and then back up, each couple greeted me with, "Are you having fun?" They seemed to take great pleasure from the whole experience.

I felt awkward, not because of the dance but because I felt it called attention to my weakness. My self-consciousness made it difficult to experience what the dance was designed to do—to have fun. Even with these mixed feeling I was pleased and deeply touched. Since then, Bob has written four more "Marjorie Dances" and has taught them to various groups of people in multiple locations.

What Bob observed was that people can tell there is something qualitatively different about these dances. It isn't that they are simple. Some of them are unusual, since they are structured differently from most contra dances. Bob designed the women's role to allow for a few moments of rest during the dance, whereas many modern contra dances keep the women moving throughout the dance.

We concluded that what I had regarded as a weakness, my continued paralysis in my right leg and foot, has helped produce dances with a strange grace. As we worked to find what would feel best for me, he created patterns of dancing that worked for me and for others too. The "Marjorie Dances." Strange grace, indeed.

Healing is Never Finished—2016

I was knocked off balance by an over-friendly dog. Flying through the air, I landed on the ground after a four-foot fall from a porch. Swelling stretched from my tailbone to my neck. Heat and ice packs were my constant companions. It could have been much worse; I was very lucky not to have broken my back or neck.

Some days were better than others, and self-care took on a different meaning; getting my hair brushed was a major accomplishment, fixing a simple breakfast was difficult. My husband's faithful support eased the hours spent "on ice."

During that healing time I managed two very short walks to the edge of the lake. Then, one morning, life felt a little brighter even as clouds scattered raindrops.

There has always been something about rain that is very comforting to me. Rainy days stir memories of my tropical South Florida childhood as torrential sheets of water blew past my window. Inside, I was warm and dry.

This day it hurt less to climb out of bed, so despite the light rain, or maybe because of it, I pulled on boots, grabbed my raincoat and hiking poles and stepped out. The overcast day seemed to delight the migrating waterfowl that visit Silver Lake in spring and fall; they ventured closer to the shoreline than usual. Thirty or more diving ducks swam just offshore. Before I could get close, these ever-wary wild birds swam off, making their way across the water to the safety of the island in the middle of Silver Lake.

The mute swans that take up residence each year responded differently to my presence, moving toward, rather than away from me, hoping for a handout. Disappointed, since I had nothing for them, they paddled off, on their way to find something of more interest than my shiny, yellow-slickered self.

Red-winged blackbirds perched in the cattail remnants of last fall. All puffed out and wind-blown, they would soon be replaced by new growth. Much of the landscape still looks wintry. The birds tell a different story. They know that spring has arrived.

And so healing began, returning me to health just as the birds returned to Silver Lake. It often occurs faster than we might imagine, but slower than we'd like.

The rain picked up and I turned back, taking a few last glances at the lake. The swans were bullying a visiting Canada goose. Red-winged blackbirds filled our neighborhood with their raucous calls. Followed the path up the hill to my home, I felt grateful for healing at whatever speed it might occur.

Grace in Action—2016

It's been many years since I was able to hop on a bike and pedal myself down the road. That saying, "just like riding a bike" always catches me. People think riding a bike is something you can't forget how to do. Yet for some of us, because of balance issues, or other losses, riding a bike is exactly what we can no longer do. Before my life changed because of paralysis I was very active. I loved to get to walk, looked forward to swimming and felt passionate about dancing. Biking was something that was easy for me.

I am grateful the paralysis has abated to some extent, yet live with many life-changing consequences, not the least of which is my inability to balance on a bike alone. After I met my second husband, Jon, a lot began to change. He was determined to figure out how to help us enjoy bike riding together.

We tried several tandem bikes and found them difficult for me to keep my feet on the pedals. While on vacation we rented a tandem bike and I was able to pedal with ease, mistaking this for healing. I thought my ankle had become more flexible. The bike we rode on along the paved paths of Sanibel Island offered me a new sense of freedom. I couldn't wait to return from vacation to get back on the tandem we'd purchased the year before.

Back home, I soon found that my ankle had not changed at all. It was the design of the bike, a Sun brand tandem beach cruiser we'd ridden on, that was different. Our quest began to obtain one for ourselves.

Two years passed before our order was filled for this somewhat foot-forward bicycle. Since then we've modified it to make it easier for my right foot to stay on the pedal. Panniers on the back of the bike make it easier to carry ice, jackets and other needed items.

And then I fell. After allowing time for healing, we woke on a gorgeous spring morning and we wondered how I could manage on our bike. We pedaled down to the end of our street for a test run, and I felt okay. Yes! We set off to find a new bike trail.

Riding our tandem is the closest I come to feeling like I'm flying. My view from the rear seat is obstructed by Jon's broad shoulders, yet I can see and feel so much, regardless. The wind blows in my face, stone walls are visible alongside paths we ride on. Swamps, streams, rivers, ponds, and birds, offer beautiful views along the way. On this ride, we spotted a snake in the middle of the path.

We stopped, turned back, concerned that the snake would be run over as it sunned itself on the warm pavement. With little encouragement from us, the garter snake slithered off the pavement back into the nearby woods. Done—our good deed for the day.

One portion of trail skirted the edge of a pond and led into the downtown area of an old New England mill town. We spotted broken down factory buildings at the edge of the water, and Jon recalled years before when he had worked in one of those buildings. Remnants of a much more prosperous era of productive factories, these structures continue standing next to the waterway for now, although they are abandoned and derelict.

I could see all this because I had ridden along on the back of our bike. While I cannot walk long distances, after healing from the latest injury, I could pedal our bike, with support.

We often hear comments from children who think our bike is "really cool!" Adults often smile and nod as we sail by. One couple stopped to talk as we ate our lunch beside the lake. They asked how we liked our bike. I answered, "I love it." They see my smile, my joy, and assume we're having fun. Truly, it is so much more. What they are witnessing, whether they know it or not, is grace in action.

A Child Shall Lead Them

A vast gulf exists between childish behavior, and a child-like attitude. They may be opposite sides of the same coin. Childishness points to the most self-centered, unpleasant parts of ourselves. A childlike perspective opens us to moments of wonder, exploration, and taking in the world as if seen for the first time. One demands everything right now; the other recognizes that now is exactly the right time to enjoy what is in front of us.

As a parent, I was confronted with my own childishness and challenged to grow up in ways I had not anticipated, working to raise my own kids. They and other little ones have taught me the importance of honoring their wit and wonder. The difficult task of parenting pushed me to learn lessons I might never have embraced otherwise. No matter our age, it is never too late to begin seeing the world through the eyes of a child.

Watching—1998

The basic premise of the game, that summer of 1965 in South Florida, was for all of us to shut our eyes and turn around in circles in our front yard. Our goal was to keep spinning till we grew dizzy. A designated "watcher" sat on the five-foot-high brick wall that jutted a few feet out into my parents' yard. The watcher's job was to keep their eyes open and warn spinning children if they drew too close to the wall, or ventured near the street.

The designated watcher achieved this by calling out, "Go away from my voice" when we got too close to the wall. However, if we got close to the sidewalk, and thus, the street just beyond, they would call out, "Come towards my voice." If, or more correctly *when,* someone fell down, we instituted a series of stages like "yellow light" or "red light" to slow the game down and keep the fallen player from getting kicked, sat upon, or squashed. The wall provided a perfect view of the entire front yard, kept the watcher from being twirled into, and was fun to sit on. We had no lack of volunteers for the position of "watcher."

The game had no "point" unless you consider having silly fun, getting very dizzy, falling down, and making a lot of noise with friends to be a worthy goal. How we came up with our rules, or even who originated the idea has been forgotten. We played, and had fun for what felt like all summer, but was probably for just a few days.

We rotated watchers throughout the evening, and each night after dinner we started over again. We sometimes wondered why the adults didn't put a stop to it. Our shrieks and hollers filled the night air. In retrospect, our parents must have been grateful we were wearing ourselves out and that no one was fighting. As long as we stayed cheerful, our parents were quite content to let the game carry on.

We felt a wonderful sense of trust and exhilaration as we twirled, knowing that when we were in danger, one of us had eyes open, warning us away from the wall, or drawing us toward his or her voice if we got near the street. Above the silliness and shrieks, the voice of the watcher rang out, clear and strong, and we obeyed it.

I smile when I think back on that summer. Our twirling game was wild and crazy and filled with more joy than I can express. Everyone was included; we set no age limit on the fun.

With our eyes closed, kids were kids, whether we were short, tall, thin or heavy, boy or girl, friend or sibling. We had no teams, no competition, just a bunch of silly, hooting and hollering kids having fun in the relative cool of a tropical summer evening, staying out as late as we could manage. We were not bored, even when we couldn't see where we were going.

Sometimes not being able to see doesn't matter very much at all—not on a summer night with your friends. Not when there's someone on the wall calling out, "Come toward my voice."

An Unexpected Gift—2002

I felt the familiar drip at the back of my throat. It was only days
before Christmas and I had too much to do to make time for a cold. I
set out for some cough medicine. As I hurried toward the entrance of
the store, I heard the tinny clinking of a bell.

It was that time again, when bell ringers stand outside stores,
familiar red kettle beside them ready to receive donations. Some wear
Santa hats, others seem bored as they maintain their posts, yet all are
stationed in such a way that no one can slip past without making eye
contact.

Our family makes donations with deliberation, choosing the
organizations we support, so I have learned to decline more unwanted
solicitations than I can count. This day, however, I felt a sudden
anxiety about ignoring the persistent bell ringer. I averted my gaze
and slipped in the door.

Once past the bell ringer, I soon located the medicine I was
looking for and headed for the checkout counter. Braced for more
guilt as I again avoided a request for funds, I emerged into the cold air
and noticed the silence; the persistent clink of the bell was missing.

A young mother with two young boys stood next to the bell
ringer. The smaller child held the bell hostage, refusing to negotiate.
His mother knelt down next to her son, putting all her tried and true
parenting methods to the test as she tried to avoid a scene and
persuade him to "give the lady back her bell, now." The determined
aspiring musician clutched the bell, a sense of resolve in his bright

brown eyes. He had decided he needed to "help" the bell ringer; perhaps he could persuade her that the bell should go home with him? I smiled. I had been there many times myself when my own children were younger.

Rather than feeling like someone was making an unwanted demand on him, this child saw the bell ringer as a person with something wonderful to give. Confident in his innocent perception, he proceeded to act on it, reveling in the sounds the bell produced as he shook it back and forth in the brisk winter air.

Many of us, with a cynical eye, have learned to anticipate demands for our attention, time, and/or money as another weight on our already burdened shoulders. Whether the appeal is from a church, a stranger, a friend, or someone in our own family, a "no" is half out of our mouths before we hear the request. Constantly on guard, we may miss what is right in front of us.

As I walked away, the tinkling of the bell resumed; the child had relinquished the cherished instrument. The grin on the bell ringer's face told me she saw her bell in a different light. Despite the worsening cold, I found I was smiling. The jingling sound followed me to my car on that crisp, cold morning so close to Christmas. Thinking I had gone to find some relief for my common cold, because of a small child and a tinny-sounding bell, I had received a welcome, unexpected gift.

Little Hands—1998

The small boy caught my attention. He had been using the kneeling bench in the church pew as exercise equipment, much to his parents' dismay. They did their best to quiet him, but he was interested in so many things, and wasn't really disturbing anyone. He stood, knelt, looked around, and made an effort to climb under the pew. His parents were having a hard time.

Then it was time to head to the altar rail. His sturdy legs carried him right up to the front of the church, where he was able to climb the steps with confidence. He stood, waiting at the rail; he was quite short. Kneeling would have meant raising his hands over his head to receive the wafer. Kneeling next to him, I studied his little hands. On the other side of him his parents waited, palms outstretched. His cupped fingers flexed open and closed in anticipation.

Chubby fingers curled and bent at the joints. He did his best to imitate the adults around him. Our priest knelt down at eye level, then spoke the words, "The body of Jesus," and gave the boy a small wafer. As if the chalice were a wonderful glass of milk ready for dunking donuts, the child dipped the wafer into the wine, popped it into his mouth, smiled, and bounded off with his parents.

Full of mischief? Oh yes. Full of life? For sure. And yes, a little child shall lead us.

Bring the Little Ones—1998

I love sitting in the front row at church for the morning service. I'm short, and sitting farther back feels as if I am standing behind other spectators at a parade, unable to see. My view is blocked from the back pews. There is always so much to take in. I don't want to miss it.

This day children launched off the platform after going up to receive communion. Some leapt from the top step, others propelled themselves from the next one. Parents' responses varied. Some made a fruitless grab for their offspring, while others found themselves dragged along, the little ones clutching their parents' hands. A few watched with tired resignation, the consequence of recent rainy days that had kept kids indoors too much.

One child left the communion rail, rubbing his tummy and letting out a tremendous "Ahhhhh." I grinned, tickled by the transparent feelings these little ones showed for all to enjoy.

I have witnessed cartwheels performed that would not have looked out of place in a gymnastics class. One is the rule, before a parent places a hand on a small head or shoulder, though on occasion a second might get slipped in before a parent intervenes. Those adults look very tired.

One morning a girl ran up the center aisle toward the railing, all two feet of her, flopped down on her knees in imitation of the grownups who surrounding her, then threw her hands in the air, palms up, as though ready to catch the biggest beach ball anyone might throw at her. What she received was a very small wafer. She walked away with a bounce and a smile.

When it was my turn to go to the rail, I heard a "crack" next to me as I kneeled. Beside me a small child had snapped his wafer in two, the sooner to eat part of it, and still have a piece for "dipping," into the wine, what we call "intinction." A protestant church, it observes differing rituals from Catholic churches. Some later insisted I had been chuckling at the altar rail. I never reveal my sources of inspiration. My belief is that giggling in church is holy laughter.

Wiggly Children—1999

Our church's practice was to bring the children in from church school to be with their parents for the last part of the service and to take communion with their families. I understood the sentiment of this practice, yet my heart went out to the mothers who had been enjoying a few moments of calm, able to listen to a sermon without tending to their children for a few moments. The mother's faces reflected this ambivalence as their kids raced to greet them.

There was joy because I knew these mothers loved their children. I also saw them pulling back on their work overalls, as it were, and settling in to keep a rein on them for the last portion of the service.

I sat with some friends and observed the pew rack in front of us transformed into a beanie baby display case, arranged and rearranged with an intense energy that kept me smiling. My friend asked her daughter if she could please try to be less wiggly, to which her daughter replied, "I just can't." We believed her.

There was the usual racing up to the altar rail for communion, kneeling down, then standing back up four or five times before taking a flying leap and racing back to their seats. This part of the service provided for large muscle movement, and these children figured it might be their only chance for awhile. The parents knew they were outmatched and did their best to maintain their dignity. Sometimes they spotted me smiling, and that's when they had to work hard not to laugh. I couldn't help myself.

Years before, a very small, wiggly boy sat in church with me. I had made the mistake of wearing a skirt with an elastic waistband. As this boy grew restless and bored, he decided to climb up and visit me on a more eye-to-eye level. I love my children and still enjoy being near them to this day, yet as he climbed upward that day, my skirt slid lower and lower, until I feared it would drop around my ankles. I took exception to this behavior. He was quite hurt, and others near me thought I was over-reacting.

I never quite got over being almost undressed by a lively child in church. Long after my children stopped treating me as a challenging mountain to climb, I avoided wearing skirts with stretchy waistbands. Despite my distress at the time, I can now look back on it and smile.

When I see these parents shaking their heads or rolling their eyes as they struggle with their young children, I smile. I haven't forgotten. Loving, caring for, and steering these little ones is not for the faint-hearted. No, I haven't forgotten at all.

Polk-ups—1997

When my daughter was born, I pulled out the flannel blankets my mother had made for her big brother. He had outgrown them. The featherstitched, red-dots-on-white-background flannel blanket became the favored snuggly for my girl. She called it "polk-ups," not quite being able to manage "polka dots." Seeing how fond she was of her flannel blanket, I offered her the other blankets Mom had made. They too became snuggly blankets, yet the hierarchy was clear. Polk-ups was the winner, or loser, since over time it was loved to shreds.

On a difficult ride home from a family visit, my girl longed for her blanket, which was waiting for her at home. It was 1987; she was four years old and very tired. As we got closer to home, still a few miles away, her sobs grew louder. I recalled a lesson learned years before, from a book that altered my approach to parenting, *How to talk so kids will listen, and listen so kids will talk,* by Adele Faber and Elaine Mazlish. It offered concrete yet adaptable strategies for working with children to solve problems and smooth the rough edges of living. An important idea I took from this book was that when it was impossible to grant a wish in reality, try bestowing wishes in fantasy. This was a situation that begged for wish-granting fantasies. I jumped in.

"I wish we were home right now."

She responded. "We aren't there yet."

I tried again. "I wish we had a helicopter to fly you home right now."

Her sobs grew louder. I tried once more. "I wish polk-ups could fly here to us right now." And she finally got it.

She answered, "I wish the whole world was polk-ups." There was nothing left to say or wish for after that heartfelt cry. We made it home, and a small girl was soon tucked into bed with her beloved blanket. I never forgot the time that my little girl captured a longing that reached far beyond our small car driving on a back road towards home. The world would be a better place if it could offer the comfort that polk-ups provided, that feeling of arriving home and being tucked into a warm bed.

Baby Blankets—2017

When I heard that our young neighbors had had their first baby, I thought to myself, *baby blanket*. I needed to make them a baby blanket. My children were the first grandchildren on both sides of our family and were showered with gifts from their grandparents. The gifts that took on lasting meaning were the flannel baby blankets my mom made for my children. She sewed many for other children too.

Mom made curtains, bedspreads, and cloth napkins by the score, stitching up the edges so they would not unravel. She gave them out as gifts, like candy. Baby blankets were on her fun projects, delighted when she came upon cute baby flannel material that she purchased by the yard. Her first were doubled up flannel fabric, sewn inside out then turned right side out. She added decorative stitching along the outer edges to assure the blanket kept its shape. Mom made blankets for whoever needed one, and all her grandchildren received them. She often sent along blankets as gifts for people she might never meet. After she died we found a stash of them in her house, waiting in reserve for the next child who needed one.

I have made a number of this same style blanket over the years, and the process of making them always brings Mom to mind. From the moment I step out of the car to head into the fabric store, Mom is right beside me in my heart, ready to offer suggestions yet allowing me to decide for myself what fabric to choose.

As I pulled out the ironing board, I felt grateful Mom taught me to sew, and to iron. The stitching task is easier when the fabric smooth and flat, so the edges line up.

I set up the sewing machine Mom gave me, and filled the bobbin with thread. Once I began sewing, I thought of this new life I was celebrating with a gift of my time, my experience, and my prayers. Would the parents understand what went into it, other than a blanket? Perhaps not. In the giving, the creating of this simple snuggly for a young child, I had been given a gift too, of thankfulness for what has been passed down to me and what has been passed on.

May you be lucky enough to have a baby blanket tradition or something akin to it in your life. What a treasure to be part of passing on that tradition, even if the passing on is just in the telling of the story.

.

Slowing Down—2018

The daily changes in a growing child are almost invisible. Over time however, clothes become too tight, toys are discarded, words are acquired, and personality is expressed.

I've been blessed with a number of grandchildren, some of whom live quite nearby. As I write, these grands are already growing up and heading to school. There was a time, however, when life was much slower.

My daughter was home with her newborn baby. The two of them made it very easy for me to be a grandma. Both new mom and new baby were pretty laid back, content and unhurried, without a whole lot on their agenda, aside from Anna creating a stacked pile from a delivery of jumbled wood that had been dumped in their back yard. I promised to watch the baby while she worked. I didn't want her to worry.

We spent most of the day together, first getting Nicole on the floor for some tummy time to strengthen her core muscles. She was happy being on her stomach. She tried to pay attention to her surroundings, but her eyes soon glazed over, her head dropped down, and she slept.

Anna fed Nicole while I cleaned the kitchen. After lunch, we took Nicole grocery shopping. Another snooze for a weary baby. Once we returned home I suggested Anna could take care of the wood while I was there. Grandma and baby snuggled down on the couch, relaxing into each other, while Anna headed outside. Nicole grew more relaxed as time passed. She fusses every now and again; a slight change of position put her right back to sleep.

It seems I got a bit of a nap too, with a baby plastered on my chest and my arm propped up with a "boppy" nursing pillow to keep us stable and snuggly. Anna checked in often, making sure all was well, then headed back out.

I held Nicole for a good part of that day, and for the most part she slept, breathing those quick, baby breaths that seem so hurried, so urgent. And yet her body conveyed contentment, comfort, assurance. "Relax, Grandma," she seemed to say. "I'm growing as fast as I can."

She is growing so fast and helps me slow down. I am reminded that there is much to experience in the quiet, in the snuggling, as she grows a little more each day.

Not By Bread Alone

Food offers much more than simple nourishment. Sharing family recipes, cooking together, and sitting down for a meal with loved ones strengthen the bonds between family and friends. Preparing meals for family, friends or strangers, can open our hearts to the joy of giving.

Memories and stories associated with food are all part of the family connections I have sought to pass on to my children and grandchildren through the years. Taste, texture, touch, and smell combine so food memories retain a lasting hold on our hearts and imaginations.

Hunting Wild Berries—2013

One hot Sunday afternoon I sought escape from the heat at the pool. I was working that last summer of high school at a Christian camp near Atlanta, Georgia, where I was a junior counselor and life guard at the camp pool. Fellow counselors warned me I would be breaking the rules by swimming on Sunday. This was "seeking my own pleasure," which was not allowed on the Sabbath. I was puzzled, and asked what was permitted. They assured me that berry picking was all right. This sounded like work to me, another Sabbath issue, and this slippery slope felt pretty treacherous. I decided it was best to stop asking questions and rounded up some others. Berry picking companions were easy to find.

My friends and I wandered the paths of camp, containers in hand, hunting for blackberries. As we walked, we chatted, found spots of cool shade, and often encountered gobs of fruit just waiting to be picked—like found treasures. The lessons that seemed intended for me to learn were quite different than what I took away from this encounter.

As an adult I have made my own peace with how to observe a Sabbath rest, and have found that picking berries still fits in well as a Sunday activity and other days too. What began as an effort to avoid censure has grown to be one of my deepest pleasures.

In New England, where I now live, small, wild, ripe blueberries become plentiful in July, and since my family enjoys walking in the woods year-round, we keep a look-out for future harvesting sites. The woods behind our house are filled with blueberry bushes. Berries thrive in the sun, so the edges of woodlands promise the best picking.

August brings blackberries. Not as friendly as blueberries, they provide a bigger harvest when one is lucky enough to find accessible canes. We pay a price in scratched arms, prickers in fingers, and blackberry stains on clothes. But the reward is great.

I start checking the wild cranberry bogs in September, hiding in plain sight near our house. The vines grow close to the ground, unobtrusive and easy to miss even thought the ripe berries turn bright ruby-red.

Through the summer and fall, I check with berry-picking partners to coordinate outings. The journey is part of the fun, sharing stories, laughing often, and remembering trails travelled in years past.

We bend or sit to pick from the low-bush blueberries we find. Our backs thank us when we encounter high-bush berries. We stretch to reach the tallest branches, where the most berries grow. We put all our boats to use to reach berries that have been tempting us on Silver Lake's island. Showers of fruit, leaves, and twigs cascade over us as we strip everything into containers. What a fun mess.

Blackberries are more challenging. With little success, we try not to snag our skin on the thorns. Almost reachable berries tempt us. My skin and shirt and sometimes my hair are ready targets for the thorn-studded canes, which leave their marks on me regardless of my best efforts. It is difficult to ignore those tantalizing jewels that are too treacherous to reach. The birds, we know, will have their feast on what we leave behind.

Cranberries grow best where there is clay soil and poor drainage, so even if all around us is dry, the ground they grow in remains wet. I try bending to pick the low-lying fruit; back pain forces me to give in and take a seat. I emerge damp, but happy, with buckets of berries in tow.

I'm never sure if it's the fruit, or the family and friends who come with me that make these times precious. In a world in which so much is beyond our control, we are able to enjoy, just for the picking, wonderful food very close to home. I love to bake with these found treasures. But when it's hottest out, ice cream with berries will do.

My children began coming with me to pick berries when they were very young. They weren't given a choice then, with predictable results at times. The next generation has arrived, and in the sunshine, as I watch my daughter picking alongside her children, my joy is complete. Seeking my own pleasure? Guilty as charged.

Blueberry Yoga—2020

In summer I head out to my yard to pick berries in the early morning light, or after dinner when the sun goes down and the air begins to cool. It's hard for me to keep active in the heat, yet in the early morning, I laugh as I stretch and twist around the gnarled branches of bushes that have been in this yard with me for so many years. Yes, Blueberry Yoga, that's it.

I bend, stretch, and reach, dragging the flexible limbs down to where I can pluck ripened fruit from the branches and drop them into my bowl. As I move amongst the branches I study the fruit, searching for dark purple berries and allowing the pink-tinged fruit to remain in the sunshine to sweeten some more.

Some years we're lucky—no late cold snaps to freeze the tender flowers in spring, lots of spring rain, and loads of hot weather and sunshine through the summer. The gypsy moths sometimes take a vacation for a year, or at least they don't chew every leaf off the bushes as has happened in the past. A reprieve, for sure.

Often the lack of summer rain requires me to offer the plants extra water. I get out early or late in the day to shower the ground around the bushes, feeding the berries with life-giving moisture. Blueberries love hot weather. Me, not so much. I left Florida years ago for cooler New England for many reasons, not the least of which was that before long summer in New England passes and I can once again feel more like a person.

I ate few berries growing up in suburban South Florida, mostly Surinam cherries off our neighbor's hedges, and guava fruits from the same neighbor's tree in their back yard. I discovered the joys of picking wild blackberries the summer I spent at a church summer camp outside Atlanta. We had as many wild blackberries as we could eat right alongside the paths of the camp. Heaven, for sure.

Soon after arriving in New England for college, I discovered wild blueberries in nearby wooded areas. After I married, berry picking became a summer priority for me and my family. When my children were small, I took them with me on walks and they soon agreed that it was fun to hunt for berries. My son could spot blueberry bushes along roadsides as we drove in the car, and he was sure to point out to me where we should hunt for berries in the coming year.

When we moved to our home near the lake in 1981, one of my first priorities was to order blueberry plants, and we installed twelve bushes at the back of our yard. They had several strikes against them from the very beginning. Large oaks shaded much of the area, reducing available sunshine. Although the bushes grew taller, they refused to set fruit. My young children had limited space in which to ride their bikes. The bushes were, for the most part, run over by energetic kids as they circled our house, mowing down one blueberry bush after the next. Of the original twelve, only three survive today.

These days, my children have grown and have given me with wonderful grandchildren. The yard is quieter. We removed a number of the trees that were too close to the house, and miracle of miracles, the remaining blueberry bushes, barren for so many years, blossomed and began to bear fruit. Joy!

Since we made room for more sunshine, some years have brought hordes of gypsy moths, stripping the plants bare and weakening them. Somehow, the bushes have survived. We have had dry springs in which few flowers managed to set fruit. In the midst of a global pandemic, with such gloom and concern in the air, my blueberry bushes outdid themselves bearing fruit.

With the arrival of warmer weather I wandered out several times a day, communing with my berry bushes. The few raspberry canes in the yard bore more fruit than usual too, and the blackberry canes were covered with fruit until a local catbird developed a taste for the juicy berries. He left us some, just not the harvest we usually get from these thorn-studded canes.

We protected from bird predation the largest blueberry bushes, draping them in netting supported by strong wooden frames that should last a number of years. The smaller bushes I planted in more recent years did not fit under the protective frame. I figured that giving the birds a portion of the harvest was the least we could do.

Having blueberries of different varieties allows the harvest to continue from late June into August, with berries for breakfast many mornings, fruit for pies, muffins, scones, and fruit crisps. We indulged again and again in my favorite fresh berry pie, a recipe we only make when the berry harvest is plentiful. The first summer in which we slow-walked through the pandemic, I made a huge dent in what some have called my pie deficit, a family joke. My husband swears I promised, when we married some fifteen years ago, to make him a pie a week. The pie deficit in our house is pretty serious.

Here's my favorite berry pie recipe, passed on to me years ago from a You Pick strawberry farm in Medway, Massachusetts. It is no longer a farm, but remains as open space.

Fresh Berry Pie

For 9" pie:

Bake single-shell pie crust, let cool.

I use the *Joy of Cooking* basic single-crust pastry recipe.

4-5 Cups berries

I've used strawberries, blueberries, or combination blue, black, raspberries, and strawberries—they're all wonderful.

2 Tbs. lemon juice

1 Cup sugar (I tend to reduce to half a cup of sugar.)

2 Tbs. cornstarch

Crush 2-3 cups of berries, stir in lemon juice, cornstarch, and sugar. Cook over medium heat until thickened, stirring constantly until the mixture is shiny. Cool slightly. Spread remaining fresh-washed berries, uncrushed, in baked pie shell, then pour berry "pudding" over fresh, uncooked berries. Chill, serve with whipped cream or ice cream, or simply eat unadorned.

Joy in baking bread—1998

I was reading a book by Julia Cameron, *The Artist's Way.* In the book she urged her readers to do something that would bring them joy. I accepted the challenge, but I was stumped wondering what would bring me joy. The barrier of "not driving" reared its ugly head, taunting me. *You can't go anywhere by yourself, unless it's with someone else driving you there.* This was in the long years after I had become ill, and my neurological symptoms made it unsafe for me to drive. A walk along the lake was possible, but that was something I did often, not something I had forgotten, or wished to do and hadn't let myself enjoy.

A thought kept intruding itself: *Why don't you make some bread?* This felt too simple. It didn't fit the parameters of what I had set out to do for myself. It would take all day! In the midst of my resistance, a voice inside me answered, *So what?* I had little to say in response, still unsure if this was what real Joy was about.

I had gone on my weekly grocery run with my friend, Carolle, whose faithfulness in helping me shop every week for seven years is another story of grace. I picked up some baking yeast just in case I decided that bread-making was the stuff of Joy. I kept thinking of all the reasons why it wouldn't be fun, or that the bread would not rise.

All through that evening, I kept wondering what kind of bread I might make. The idea felt better and better. The next day was my dad's birthday. It all began to make sense. Dad had been the ultimate bread baker in our family while I was growing up.

I woke and organized the ingredients for bread making, an activity that felt familiar as from another time. I recalled my dad getting up every Saturday morning throughout my childhood, finishing breakfast, and setting up all his equipment and ingredients and "clearing off a space on the counter," as he so often said. I often wandered through, asking to help and was always invited to take part in his simple routine. He would hand me a piece of dough, and we kneaded our dough until it was shiny and ready for rising.

As he worked the bread with his strong hands, we chatted. It didn't matter what we talked about as there always seemed to be something to say as we stood side by side. Even if I didn't feel like helping, I often kept him company, and he seemed glad to have me or others stop by.

My parents loved to retell a family story of the day Mom brought home a friend from church, a older woman we all enjoyed. Mom had some things to do, so she asked my dad, "Could you entertain Jean for awhile?" Dad's response was to make bread for her.

As she sat on the kitchen chair, Dad narrated his process, keeping her in stitches. He never measured anything, and poked fun at himself by pointing out how he was going to put in two cups of milk. He then poured some water from the faucet into the bowl, then added a scoop of powdered milk. The bottle of cooking oil was "butter." Everything he added was supposed to be one thing, yet was really something else, all presented with a twinkle in his eye. Jean could hardly stay in the chair she laughed so hard.

Mom couldn't believe what she saw when she came back: indeed, Dad had kept Jean entertained by baking bread. In fact, he did it every week for us, without ever calling it entertainment.

When Dad's bread came out of the oven we could never wait to eat it. The yeasty smell of fresh-baked bread drew us into the kitchen to enjoy the savory treat. We squashed many a loaf because we would not wait for the bread to cool, sawing off slices right out of the oven (bread collapses a bit when sliced too soon!). No need for toasting to melt the butter, just hot bread and butter. As many of us as were home flocked to the kitchen, ready for a piece. Both heels of the bread were awarded to whoever got there first. Before we knew it, the first loaf had disappeared.

Dad would stare at the remaining bread and sigh. "That's why I always have to make more than one. You all eat the first before I can blink. At least there's more for sandwiches." There was, but it was never quite as good as those first warm slices, fresh out of the oven.

My bread had a texture unlike than Dad's, but was quite edible. Thanks, Dad. Wish you were here to help, and in so many ways, you are. The joy is here, too. Quiet joy. Different from those Saturday mornings, yet in many ways just the same.

Traveling in Time with Food—2018

My grandgirl and I had already spent time making salads, baking bread, and making cookies, but we had never made banana bread together. She and I had a free afternoon and I had bananas in the freezer just waiting to be transformed into banana bread, a wonderful treat for breakfast and other times too.

I reached for my mother's recipe book, published in 1949, and given to Mom as a wedding gift. Many recipe books have directions for how to make banana bread, yet I like how this one turns out. It must be the buttermilk.

As I opened the recipe for banana bread, Nicole stared at the page and commented, "It looks like a lot of the ingredients fell here!" We laughed, and I told her that Florida Grannie and Florida Grampie (as she referred to her great-grandparents in Florida,) used this book many times. My memories of baking banana bread are associated with my dad. I suspect he had something to do with the "decorations" on the page.

We had soon assembled the ingredients. I helped Nicole measure flour, baking soda, baking powder, sugar, butter, and buttermilk. We paid extra attention to the teaspoon measures and practiced using fractions as we worked. She cracked an egg into a separate bowl, I extracted a few stray egg shells, and on we went.

With each step, Nicole asked questions. What joy to pass on simple kitchen knowledge to my growing grandgirl, who soon would approach my own height. She wanted a turn with the nut chopper and took great delight in whacking away at the nuts to pulverize them before dumping them into the bowl along with everything else.

The bananas were different issue. She was willing, just not quite sure what to expect since the frozen, now thawed bananas were squishy, almost slimy in texture. She soldiered on and all the bananas ended up in the bowl.

Once everything was mixed and into the oven, she had more questions. One stopped me. "What will you do with this book when you don't need it any more, Grandma?"

Ah, she is getting old enough to grasp that none of us lives forever, even if that's not what she said. I admitted I hadn't thought much about it. "Would you like it someday?" I asked. She nodded and hugged me.

Passing on family stories happens in many ways. Sometimes baking together and letting the conversation flow as our hands are busy are the most natural places to start. Making room for the next generation in our kitchens is a real gift—for the younger generation as well as for those of us who have been around for awhile. For those interested, here's the recipe:

Banana Bread Recipe

Mix dry ingredients:

2 cups white or wheat flour

½ tsp. baking powder

½ tsp. baking soda

¼ tsp. salt

Then cream together:

¼ cup sugar and

¼ cup butter

Add 1 egg

Add dry ingredients to wet ingredients, then

Add 2/3 cup mashed bananas

Add 3 Tbs. buttermilk (I use powered buttermilk and add the powder with three Tbs. of water)

Add ½ cup chopped walnuts

Place mixture in a greased bread pan and bake at 350 degrees for about 50 min.

Coconut Traditions—2015

We have many choices of activities to do around the holidays, and making time for family traditions is pretty high on my list of "things to do." This day's to-do list included making coconut candy with a grandgirl and her mom.

My parents made two types of coconut candy when I was growing up. The original family recipe was for sugared coconut. Toasted coconut candy was a recipe my parents developed later. For the sugared variety, place prepared coconut, detailed below, in a large pot with sugar, one cup of sugar per coconut, with no water added. Stir constantly until all the sugar is absorbed. This was the original recipe my dad's parents came up with after encountering on their travels the sugared coconut candy in a shop in San Francisco.

Dad worked for the telephone company, and part of his job as a forecaster—projecting growth in then-rapidly expanding South Florida—was to drive around counting house foundations as a way to quantify where the biggest need for new telephone lines would be. "Counting houses" is what Dad called it.

We were always thrilled to learn Dad had been out doing this, since he often managed to bring home five or six coconuts he'd found on his tours around Broward County. As northerners throw out piles of leaves in the fall, many people in South Florida regarded coconuts as yard waste and placed them by the curb to be picked up with the rest of their trash. Dad stopped when he spotted the nuts and set them onto the back seat of his car. We kids were enlisted to help turn this "trash" into treasure: the beloved coconut candy.

My own preference is toasted coconut, the recipe my parents devised after they were married. I couldn't say when I first made it. In my family as I was growing up, it was just something we did every year.

First the outer husks, which grocery shoppers will never see, had to be removed. These green husks are more than twice as large as the inner nut, and are the stuff floor mats are made from—coir. We drove two shovel tips back to back into the top of the husk, then pulled the handles together, prying the thick outer covering away from the inner shell, which is what you will find in grocery stores when buying fresh coconuts.

My children grew up in Massachusetts. Despite not living in the tropics like I had, they learned the secrets of making coconut candy, and year after year we bought coconuts at the grocery store to make the candy for Christmas gifts.

I always check to be sure there's lots of coconut "water" still inside the nut. Shake it—you'll hear the liquid slosh around inside the nut. Its presence makes the difference between an edible and inedible coconut. This same important coconut water will also make a mess if you don't drain it out before you crack open the nut!

When my daughter and granddaughter arrived, I got out the hammer and screwdriver—essential tools in this process. Nicole thought using a hammer and screwdriver in the kitchen was pretty cool. We made holes in two of the three "eyes" (dark spots at the top of the nut) of each of our two coconuts, then drained the water before we moved to the next step. I never liked the taste of coconut water when I was a child, and despite some people's enthusiasm for it (I see it bottled in grocery stores now) I still pass on drinking it.

We then wrapped each drained nut in a plastic bag to ensure no sharp chunks would go flying once we started hammering. After placing the wrapped nut on the floor, Anna and Nicole each took some good swings and soon had the nuts open, ready for the next step.

My parents taught us an easy trick for getting the white meat out of the coconut shell. We placed the broken pieces on a baking tray, set it in a 350-degree oven for about fifteen minutes, let the pieces cool, and then popped the meat out with a dull knife. Easy! Next, that inedible brown skin on the outer portion of the meat—not tasty—needed to be removed. The vegetable peeler helped make short work of removing the brown, outer skin, then a quick rinse of the white meat, and we were ready for... more work.

Within about an hour we had transformed two coconuts into a tray full of coconut meat, sliced into half-inch wide curls ready for toasting. We used a vegetable peeler to get just the right thickness. A teaspoon of salt per coconut, sprinkled lightly over the entire shallow tray of coconut was all the seasoning this treat required. A 250-degree oven did the rest of the work, and my kitchen timer reminded us to stir the coconut every twenty minutes or so. After about an hour, the tray was almost completely toasted, with hints of the white meat still showing amidst the golden-brown curls.

Nicole was only six at the time, so her interest in the process flagged. We found other things for her to peel while Anna and I continued the process. My daughter noted that it had been years since we had made coconut candy. Why now? Because it was time to ensure another generation knew how to make this special treat. It was also a chance for the next generation to hear the stories of my dad and his family traveling from Minnesota to South Florida, seeking a place where Dad's father could feel better, despite suffering from severe arthritis. In Miami they found not only a climate where my grandfather was more comfortable, they also discovered tropical delights such as coconuts and began what has become a tradition in our family.

When it comes to Christmas presents, making time to do things together with those you love is right at the very top of my list of precious gifts. My heart was full, my kitchen smelled wonderful, and a tradition was passed on to another generation.

Hands-on Memory Making—2016

Pie-making was on the agenda, as was putting together the cranberry relish. My grandgirl was available and willing, so I got her off the school bus and brought her straight to my kitchen so we could get to work.

We've made pies together before—she knows the drill and is passionate about pumpkin pie. We would be making apple pies too, but the pumpkin pie was the priority. We pulled out the cans of pumpkin and evaporated milk, plus eggs, and spices. We decided to get this done first since our other projects would be more labor intensive. I had mixed up several batches of pie dough the day before so it would be chilled and ready to use.

Once the pumpkin pie was in the oven we tackled the apple pies. I have a special brown-handled knife I've used since my kids were small, a cheese knife really; it only cuts hard things, not soft things like fingers. The knife works great on apples, carrots, and potatoes, but is not good for stringy foods such as celery. My children knew they could be part of the cooking process once they learned how to handle this real, but not so sharp, brown-handled knife. My grands now enjoy using it too, and are happy that they have can handle a real knife in the kitchen.

Nicole is getting the hang of rolling out dough and has fun playing with leftover pastry. On this day when we had four pies scheduled, there was no shortage of chances to practice with Grandma's rolling pin.

After slicing the apples, the last step before baking the pies was to coat the top of the pie crusts with plain yogurt. It works as well as milk or an egg wash in making the baked crust crisp and shiny. Such fun for a grandgirl to dive into a dish of yogurt and get messy with Grandma.

Once the pumpkin pie was baked and the apple pies were in the oven, we assembled everything for the cranberry relish. The most essential tool is the meat grinder I grew up using. It's a once-a-year piece of equipment, perfect for young (and older) folks to use to grind apples, oranges, and cranberries into a crushed, ground up mass of delicious relish. My kids were always ready to help with this task when they were younger. When my son was here a few years ago for Thanksgiving, he dove right into the job, showing his young son how much fun it was to turn the hand crank and see the berries, apples, and oranges transformed into relish.

More often it was my daughter who took on grinding duties when she was younger. This day was a grandgirl's turn.

The relish was made, the pies were golden brown and baked, and Grandma was pretty pooped. Nicole took only a few breaks, and one of her breaks was to clean up the dishes, which provided a great excuse for water play. We laughed about her attending "Camp Grandma." Yes, I took pictures. My hope was that she was also storing up memories—memories of helping, of having fun, of being an essential part of her extended family. Memories of those who have gone before us, cooking, baking, grinding, and caring are an important part of what family is all about.

The Strength of Family and Friends

We humans were not created to live alone. Living together, however, can be hard! Despite our social nature, we all need time alone. Rubbing the rough edges off one another is what family seems to do best. Truth-tellers who are life-long friends or who enter our lives for a season bring that same grace to our lives.

The other side of the powerful force for good that family and friends offer is that these same people can have a negative impact on our lives. Learning to set limits, to respond creatively, and to maintain our boundaries can take a lifetime of practice. For better or worse, our family and friends make a difference in our lives

Rainbows—2011

A Christmas gift from my cousin became the foundation of a small collection I've added to over the years. It is an elongated glass prism, which was at one time part of a crystal chandelier.

I visited a friend's home and saw her windows strung with hundreds of glass prisms. I asked, "How do you hang them?" Dental floss. So simple, and not something I would have thought of. My gift soon dangled in my kitchen window, strung up with floss to catch each morning's light, casting rainbows all about my small kitchen.

Over time I found other pieces to add to my collection. Family and friends gave them to me. When my mother died I found a box filled with multiple prisms, much like the original one hanging in my kitchen, parts of an unknown chandelier. I claimed several to hang with the others. When a dear friend moved away I gave a prism from my window to her, a token of our friendship. Others soon filled the empty space in my window.

When my husband did some work in our kitchen we took down the fragile glass pieces, both for safekeeping and because he was altering the kitchen walls. I tucked them all in a box lined with packing material to protect them from breakage.

Recently my daughter gave me a small prism "for your collection." It needed hanging, so when my friend visited, I suggested she help me return the glass pendants to the light. Sue loves projects like this and is comfortable using tools of all kinds. We located a drill and measuring tape, and before long seven cup hooks were installed, ready for the hanging glass pieces that would create rainbows.

I had many more than seven prisms to choose from. I found the original gift that began my collection, put it with the newest addition from my daughter, then chose five more to fill the window. Sue looked at the leftover prisms and said, "I'm visiting my dear friend soon. Could I have two identical ones, one for her and one for me, so we can each share the same rainbows?" I invited her choose some, then wrapped them with care for their journey.

In summer I must rise early to catch these rainbows. In winter the scattered light dances about the east side of my house as the prisms take their time shining their light across the kitchen and adjoining rooms. As I stand at the sink preparing food, clearing up from a meal, or simply looking out at birds visiting my feeder, I delight in sunshine turned into scattered rainbows cast thither and yon through these many-facetted crystals.

My kitchen is once again filled with reflected light. What began as a single piece of cut glass has become a much-loved collection and has given blessings far beyond what I could have imagined.

We might think we can control what we give to others. In reality we have no say over the results. This as it should be, and is part of the risk, the magic of sharing. All gifts offer possibility, whether you ever learn what happens later or not.

Echoes Through the Generations—2018

When I saw the photo, my first thought was "That's my son." I was assured the young man in the photo, standing in the dirt road, was actually my grandfather Glen.

I'd never met this grandfather, who died before I was born, and yet, I knew that stance. It was so familiar because my own son often assumed the same pose as his great-grandfather, arms crossed at the waist, looking thoughtful, listening intently, or taking in his surroundings.

This same son grew up hearing stories of Glen, my father's father. One of my dad's favorite stories to tell was of the cherry table his father Glen rescued from a farmer's yard in Quebec back in the 1940s. Each summer Glen and my grandmother Marjorie (my namesake) traveled to Canada in search of antique furniture for him to refinish in his workshop. Somehow they came across a farm in which the chicken coop's walls were constructed from a cherry wood table. Presumably legs and all were still attached. Glen offered to buy the table from the farmer, but his offer was refused. "Nope, I need the chicken coop." Glen offered to build the farmer a new chicken coop. Then could he purchase the cherry table? They struck a deal, and the cherry wood table, presumably in pretty tough shape, returned with my grandparents to South Florida and was lovingly restored to its former glory.

The boards of this table are wide, the gleam of the wood now bright, and the grain is beautiful. Over the years many family meals were eaten at this table, and after my grandparents died, my aunt and uncle enjoyed it in their home and used it for the many dinners they hosted for family and friends. When they sold their house they were unable to take the large table with them to their new living quarters. My son said his family would be glad to have the table at their farm in Tennessee.

We visited my son and daughter-in-law recently and enjoyed multiple meals at this same table that was rescued from the chicken yard so many years ago. My grandchildren will now grow up hearing the story of the grandfather from years past, who had eyes to see beyond the grime of the chicken yard and understood the potential that lay underneath the grit and muck. The table was transported once again, to another generation, and back to the farm. The table and the stories that lie behind had found their way home.

In another part of the farmhouse hangs the picture of this grandfather as a young man, standing as his great-grandson does so often, arms crossed in front of him, looking intently, listening closely, and taking in his surroundings.

Fluttering Rows of Hospitality—1998

Taking in the laundry from the clothesline as the sun set gave me time to listen to the sounds of our neighborhood settling down for the day. As I folded our towels and shirts, checking each for dampness, the rhythm of the evening set in.

Kids are not quiet near sunset; they are more inclined to giggle, shriek, and scream after having been let loose for some running around before turning in for the night. The basketball's thump-thump set a rhythm to all the other noises, the base drum in the neighborhood band.

I could hear the tinkling of silverware and dishes being cleaned up, a follow-up to the murmuring coming from nearby families sitting together to eat. I peered at my clothesline and saw not simply cloth napkins hanging there. I also saw a fluttering row of hospitality, reminding me of dinners shared and visits enjoyed.

Birds quiet down at this time of evening in mid-summer. Everything feels softer as the sun goes down and evening sets in.

Taking down clothes down from the clothesline. Another mindless activity, like cleaning, that allows my mind to focus on other things. As my children were growing up, bringing in clothes from the line at the end of the day gave me a front row seat for kid's accomplishments, great or small. I was a cheerleading presence when the youngest children in the neighborhood discovered the euphoria of riding a two-wheeled bike without training wheels. Their endless circles around our little dead-end street gave me the chance to acknowledge their efforts. I was available to see the ebb and flow of friendship and the arguing that threw some together while leaving others out, usually for a very brief time. After a conversation with me about nothing, they were off to the races again.

A fluttering row of hospitality. Are cloth napkins much trouble? I don't think so. They're part of everyday life around here. Cloth napkins need no ironing, can be reused from meal to meal, and are a sweet reminder of my mom's love. She was the one who made them for us.

The row of colorful pieces of fabric waving in the breeze was evidence of the multiple snacks and meals enjoyed with neighbor children. They were frequent visitors when my own kids were growing up. No, cloth napkins and all they represent are not any trouble at all.

The Pink Princess—2020

We rarely get to choose who our neighbors are. Little did I know when I moved to the house at the top of the hill overlooking Silver Lake, that I would someday hit the jackpot of caring friends who were close by when I needed them most. Some offered child care when I faced divorce court. Others gave a listening ear as I worked to figure out how to care for my family, and company through those earliest days of convalescence after surgery. The most important gift, however, was including me in neighborhood events that happened here with great frequency as my kids grew up.

Among the many memories I cherish from this time in my life was the crowning of the pink princess. Julia was the long-awaited girl in her family after a string of brothers. Despite Chris's enthusiasm for entertaining she hated to sew. I volunteered to help Julia's dreams of becoming a pink princess for Halloween come true. We went together to choose the right shade of pink fabric for her costume. As I sewed, Julia provided exacting directions for how the dress was to be put together.

The future pink princess came over to try on her costume before hemming. As she pulled the dress on over her little shoulders she began to shake. Was she cold? "No, I am so excited." Her tiara sat lightly upon her head that Halloween.

Halloween was anticipated and planned for each year. A potluck dinner was part of the fun, complete with eyeball chili, Halloweiners, and whatever other recipe we could come up with that had any connection to the day. Adults and kids together went trick-or-treating to visit neighbors along the lake, then returned to have a candy exchange. The older kids had no problem bargaining the little ones out of their chocolate bars.

As Julia grew, she jumped in as "party consultant" with her mom and me to plan events that included everyone who lived here or happened to be visiting. The undercurrent of each celebration, which in reality lasted only about fifteen minutes, was to have fun with neighbors and friends.

Chris enlisted Julia to help host tea parties. Group Easter egg dyeing classes became an annual event. Christmas called for willing children to build graham cracker gingerbread houses. Chris purchased the candy; I whipped egg whites for the edible "royal icing" that held crackers and candy in place.

Our neighborhood celebrated many holidays together until Julia and her family moved away. Chris soon fell ill with cancer and died within weeks, a loss her family and I still feel.

Julia recently married and once again she became the Pink Princess, a title she has worn with ease. Her mother's absence at the wedding brought tears of grief in the midst of joy. My presence could not make up the loss, but the bride knew I remembered. It was the wedding gift I was able to give, and had to be enough.

Celebration—2000

Against all odds, we managed to celebrate my parent's fiftieth wedding anniversary the summer of 1999. This might not seem so remarkable except that my parents had always artfully avoided any manner of celebration of their marriage since their wedding day itself, fifty years before.

We all, including my parents, got ourselves to Pensacola, Florida, where my parents had been married. Both Mom and Dad had developed illnesses that nearly kept them from making the trip that year. Overcoming the odds, we all arrived at the beach houses we'd rented only to find that we couldn't swim in Santa Rosa Sound. A major sewage spill had contaminated the water right next to where our rentals stood. To reach the Gulf of Mexico from where we stayed was a short walk across the island. The waters of the Gulf provided a welcome respite from the Florida heat.

We had tried to figure out when we could make a real celebration for my parents, but hadn't been able to see our way clear. We ran into cousins of my mother, who were also at the beach that week. They offered a place for the perfect party setting. Mom's cousins, the Rule family, own the house our grandmothers grew up in, at 619 N. Baylen Street. My parents had held their wedding reception there fifty years before.

In deference to the many of our crowd who were under the age of three, we made it a morning party. Ten o'clock. An outing to 619 (with no mention of a party) was arranged and Dad was encouraged to come. Mom needed no encouragement.

Just before we were ready to head out, Mom announced that they needed to take the camper to Ft. Pickens to dump its septic tank (a theme of the week, apparently). Since the party was to be a surprise, my brother Rob did some quick talking, suggesting that many of us were interested in the gathering, and if Mom and Dad got back to the beach house and found no one there, they should just come on over to 619. Dad remained unfazed by this. Mom began to Suspect.

Many had already arrived when I got there. The cake was set up. A beautiful, pen-and-ink family tree hung on a nearby wall. My brother, Rob and his family had put it together with effort and loving creativity. My favorite part of the family tree, shaped like a real tree, not just a staggered list of names, was that all the grandchildren's pictures were nestled atop images of mangoes suspended from the branches. I love to think of my children and nieces and nephews as mangoes.

Mom and Dad did not move quickly, and the visit to Ft. Pickens took longer than they had thought, so we had plenty of time to wander the rooms of 619, which our great-grandfather had built for his bride in 1894. We admired the stunning fireplaces, built-in drawers that went from floor to ceiling, nooks and crannies, and old bathroom fixtures. My memories from brief visits as a child were of the kitchen elevator and the porch swing. The elevator was the favorite of the many children at this party.

The Happy Couple finally arrived, and Mom was quick to figure out that the sea of blue-green "Beachnuts" family reunion t-shirts could mean only one thing. In anticipation of the expected photo opportunity, everyone wore that year's reunion shirt.

Greeted with smiles and cheers, Mom and Dad entered 619 to be duly honored. It was about time. Cameras started snapping, directions for who should be in group pictures were called out, and Mom had a story. As she stood on the third step of the gracefully winding staircase, she recalled how she had stood on that very step to throw her wedding bouquet, upon the direction of the photographer who insisted she stand there. Mom had wanted, dreamed, of standing at the top of the staircase. She complied with the photographer's wishes for the picture's sake. And then someone had stepped in front of the camera at just the wrong moment, so the picture was spoiled anyway. She hadn't forgotten.

The party was brief, and perfect. We stood on the porch to take group pictures, forty-plus family and friends jammed as close together as we could. I was squeezed towards the middle and found myself next to Mom. Her eyes brimming with tears, she turned to me and confessed, "I hoped something like this might happen. It's really nice that it did." It *was* nice, and a lot more.

Shared Adventures—2000

Having lived with my parents till I was seventeen, I'd seen them under less than ideal circumstances at times. Being a parent myself, I have grown to understand the joys and pitfalls of sharing one's life with others. Especially when others are watching our every move, and quite willing to point out the failures and disappointments that inevitably occur in day-to-day living, there is no way to hide who we really are.

My parents grew up and lived in Florida. Since their grandchildren were, for the most part, here in New England, they made it a habit to come visit us each summer.

When we left Florida at the end of the family reunion week, Mom announced that they were all coming to New England! She pointed out that with so many of us around, there had been little time to really be with one another. She was right. Thus, they made their way, once more, on their annual summer pilgrimage.

During their visit at my house I had a meeting at church one night, and my parents were concerned that I was too tired to drive myself. Dad was going to drive me, and then Mom decided she would go along for the ride too.

They dropped me off, and as they prepared to back out I noticed, through the window, that they had stopped and both had gotten out of the car. Since it was raining, I thought this was sort of unusual.

Mom saw me looking through the window, poked her head in and announced, "We're going to see if we can find any birch logs." I shrugged. Sure. Don't everyone's parents go traipsing through the rain at 7:30 at night, looking for birch logs?

Before long, Mom returned to the window with a big smile on her face. She assured me, "We found what we were looking for!" Off they headed for home.

After they left, I found myself thinking about them. About how different from each other they seemed to those who didn't know them. Dad, so quiet and reserved. Mom, anything but quiet, anything but reserved.

Mom was usually up for all sorts of adventures, while Dad was much more inclined to stay home and read quietly. Then I pictured the two of them tromping through the woods behind our church.

I was sure Mom spotted what looked like birch trees. "Let's go look." She got a gleam in her eye when she had an idea. Dad, truly a good sport, climbed out of the car to go with her. Mom kind of bounced, while Dad followed along with a twinkle in his eye.

One thing my parents loved almost more than anything was a quest. My sister-in-law had asked them to find her some birch bark, so she could help her children, whom she was home-schooling, to build a birch bark canoe. A little one, nothing huge....

They'd succeeded in their quest. One large birch log, already cut down, "just waiting" as my dad said, "for us to pick it up."

Watching them set off on this simple adventure, I recognized that I was seeing, right in front of me, a picture of love. Joy in the simple. Shared adventure. And hanging in there, even when the going sometimes felt very, very rough.

Joy and Grief—2000

Within months of that anniversary celebration for our parents, and their summer visit to New England, my brothers and sisters, all five of us, had gathered again, this time at my parents' house, along with our children, cousins, and our aunt and uncle. Mom had died after a very brief bout with cancer. We wanted to be with our dad, and to be together.

The house was not huge, yet we borrowed mattresses, used our parents' camper, and somehow squeezed nineteen of us in. There was great comfort in just being there.

With any death come countless details—phone calls to answer, people to pick up at airports, visitors to welcome. The night before Mom's memorial service, it was just my brothers and sisters and me. The spouses had gone to bed, the younger children too. My children, the oldest, remained in the living room, and two of our dearest cousins sat nearby as Mom's five children gathered in a circle. We were conscious that we might never have a time just like it again.

We had decided to invite people to tell stories about Mom at her memorial service, and began talking about what stories we might tell. As the evening before the service grew late, we got reacquainted with each other. We have a rather wide age span between us, and many events had happened that some of us had not been aware of. I, the middle one, was amazed by all I'd missed. Laughter punctuated many of our tales.

We agreed not to tell some of what we talked about that night the next day at Mom's funeral. These were stories, as one of us put it, "from another lifetime." But we heard them that night, together, in my parents' living room. My teenagers grinned, remaining quiet, enjoying their elder's awkward stories of days gone by.

We heard about youthful adventures and Mom's tolerance, nay, encouragement, even delight, in our exuberances. How Dad always tried to draw the line and Mom lobbied for us to be given "one more chance." My vehemently anti-gun sister discovered that Mom had used one of this sister's forgotten embroidery projects to sew a cloth case for our brother's BB gun. She was shocked—shocked! We laughed and laughed.

There were many stories of Pensacola, and our visits to our grandmother's beach house. Memories stirred of time spent each summer at the beach growing up. What hard work, and probably not much fun, for Mom to get us all packed. The drive from our house to the beach house took about thirteen hours, even longer before the highways were improved.

Our youngest brother recalled an event at the beach. He was quite small, seven or eight, when Mom awakened him one night. She brought him out to Santa Rosa Sound to see the glowing phosphorescence in the water. That mystical green glow of tiny sea creatures would light up when touched either by the gentle waves or by those who swam into them.

Rob marveled that Mom would get him out of bed in his underwear, take him down to the dock and encourage him to get in the water at night to experience the magic. A gift to a small boy. As he said the next day at her service, "Mom didn't follow all the rules. She did things because they were fun."

The clock was nearing midnight when we heard Dad come down the hall. He'd gone to bed hours before and we realized we might have been disturbing him. We all turned as he came into the room.

He stood at the edge of our circle, refraining from joining us. With tears in his eyes he said, "You don't know what a gift this is, to see you all enjoying each other, laughing together. It makes me feel that what your mother and I tried to do worked—that you love each other and can have fun together. Don't let me interrupt, you just go on." He returned to his room, to the bed he had shared with Mom for over fifty years.

We told many stories the next day, and did not, as promised, tell others. We felt a deep joy hearing, from people we didn't know, of the other life Mom had had beyond our immediate and extended family.

As the stories came to a close, Mom's voice—the voice of the one who had a story for every occasion—was silent. Her silence reinforced our loss. The gifts she gave … they continue on.

Forging Connections—2015

Each generation and every family has unique life situations. Some families I know live within multiple generations under one roof. Others live on separate coasts and have to squeeze in limited visits when possible. My own children offer a similar contrast—one family lives right here in town, while the other lives a three-hour plane flight away on a farm that ties them down, making return visits to see us difficult to manage.

School vacations offer some special three-generation family time for us—my daughter, who works full-time, had taken the week off, making outings with grands easier for me to enjoy. I got to appreciate how hard my daughter works with her kids, and what fun she has with them.

The grands know that Grandma likes to get outside, and when I pick them up on an afternoon they will often ask, "Where are we going today, Grandma?" We were blessed with some sunny days during one vacation week and picked a couple of places to venture out to for a "hike." This is a term I use guardedly, since David, then three, while a sturdy fella, wearied quickly, and my own "hiking" means walking on clear paths with solid footing. With snow still on the ground I needed to pick places where parking lots had been plowed. Because of the age of my fellow "hikers," it helped to have a playground as the reward after venturing out on a trail.

The snow and ice near the pond at Choate Park in Medway, Massachusetts, near where we live, made for a challenging outing.

Grands found stone walls to climb on and jump off. We found the path to be icy, so after traveling a short distance, we turned back and headed for the promised playground.

The next day we picked a different hiking spot, Hopedale Parklands. The trails there were easier to navigate. It appeared the parks crew in Hopedale had been out on the trail, trimming trees, and the path was clear of snow for the most part. The trails were perfect for sliding and slopping along in snow boots, and running about.

Boulders alongside the path made for great climbing for the grands; we came across a rock shelf along the trail that was a perfect natural slide. David pushed us to continue on to the stone bridge, another exciting part of this trail system. Fast-fading sunlight forced us to choose between a longer walk and time at the playground. The playground option won.

There are no "right" ways to be a grandparent. It doesn't matter what you do together, as long as you do something, and everyone ends up most of the time smiling. As my daughter chased her little ones around the swings and slides, I grew tired just watching them, yet felt great joy witnessing them stretch their strong limbs, balance on the playground equipment, and herd each other down the slides. It was just one way to build memories, forging connections between generations. I consider myself lucky to have this time with my own children and with the next generation too.

Old Letters as Time Machines—2012

I never realized that doing the work of preserving a family legacy—the photos that tell stories, documents, letters, and the tales themselves—could actually be a powerful time machine. My dad taught me this, as he taught me so much else.

I was ready to wrap up Dad's memoir when my sister handed me a box of family papers. In the box I found the courtship letters Dad had written every day to my mother as she finished her last year of college. She saved each one. The couple lived hours apart, saw little of each other during this time, and were deeply in love.

I brought what Dad had written and asked if he was willing to include them in his memoir. He expressed trepidation: he had no idea what he might have said sixty years before. Mom had been dead twelve years, and he had never stopped mourning her loss.

When I met him for breakfast the morning after I had handed him the letters, his eighty-nine-year-old face shone. He thanked me for bringing them. Then he said, "I stayed up till midnight reading these, and it felt like I was sitting there writing to her, just like it was sixty years ago." He handed me the letters "for safekeeping." They had served their purpose.

With his blessing I transcribed and included these letters in his completed memoir, which Dad was able to hold before he died. One theme flowed throughout the letters from that twenty-six-year-old man to his bride-to-be: We're apart for now, but soon we'll be together, as we were meant to be.

Weeks after his book was completed Dad died, and was indeed with Mom again, as they were meant to be. Those letters had been an unexpected time machine, transporting him back to when he was young and deeply in love with the woman he would be married to for fifty years.

There is no guarantee where the time machine of documenting a legacy might take you. If you're very lucky, you may be taken to a time of great joy—or possibly great pain. Some stories you may be willing to share with your loved ones, while you may choose to keep others to yourself. You'll never know, however, unless you're willing to take the first step

Lessons Learned

Time and distance have offered me some perspective. Occasionally I have gained sudden insights. Some events have been difficult to make peace with. Practicing patience has been essential, though rarely welcome. With the benefit of hindsight I am now able to see that much good has come out of what felt at times to be hopeless situations.

Writing this book has taken me close to thirty years. Rather than try to explain everything I have learned, I'd rather tell you some stories. Take what you need from them, and leave the rest.

Lessons must be relearned sometimes. That in itself is worth remembering.

Journey of Faith—2016

(First published in Christine Keddy's blog, Missistine.com)

When I was ten, I discovered on my parents' bookshelf a ten-volume set of books encompassing both Old and New Testament stories. Once I began reading, I couldn't put them down. Written in a somewhat old-fashioned manner, with plenty of moralizing provided in a summary at the end of each story, I absorbed the stories and ignored the moralizing. The books graphically portrayed the characters that populated the books of Genesis, the Exodus, the adventures of the Israelites, the prophets, and the promise of the longed-for Messiah. Much was left out—these stories were aimed at children—but what was there created a foundation for my understanding of scripture, God's way of working in the world, and his promises.

Because of my reading, I was well-versed in the Bible stories taught in Sunday School at the Presbyterian church we attended. I became an insufferable know-it-all. My mother taught my fifth-grade Sunday School class, and the children in the class accused her of giving me all the answers.

In high school I discovered C.S. Lewis's "The Screwtape Letters." I smiled in recognition as the demon mentored his hapless apprentice tempter, describing with such accuracy and insight human behaviors and vulnerabilities. Lewis's books about Narnia transported me to a place I'd never imagined, while confirming spiritual truths I had grown to understand and claim as my own.

College took me from Florida to New England, to attend Gordon College, where I hoped to gain some grounding in more intellectual Christian thought. I spent two years there, made some life-long friends, and attended challenging seminars with professors who lived godly lives and asked difficult questions

Thomas Merton's "The Seven Story Mountain," a Trappist monk's memoir of coming to faith in the Roman Catholic tradition, was eye-opening to me as an adult and first-time mother. I'd never encountered the concept of contemplation or mysticism, especially within the context of the historical Christian church. The more I read, the more Merton's writings resonated with me. How strange. Me, a young married woman nursing my first child. What could I have in common with a celibate Trappist monk, a Roman Catholic, living a vow of silence? I'd spent my entire life attending Protestant Churches and agreeing with the tenets of the Christian faith as seen through the eyes of the Protestant Reformation. Yet, his experiences opened my eyes to new ways of thinking about my own faith. Merton introduced me to an entirely new world of Christian thought.

At twenty-nine, I faced divorce and the need as a single mother to care for my two very young children. The teachings I'd grown up with in Presbyterian and Baptist churches I'd attended contradicted the choices I faced. "Real Christians don't get divorced," was a not-so-subtle message I'd absorbed through those years. "Divorce is from hardness of heart. Turn the other cheek, preferring others rather than yourself." Everywhere I turned in my daily scripture readings the message seemed to be to obey my husband, who was urging me to abandon my children, to get out of his and my children's lives. Feeling beaten down, I was sorely tempted to cede to his demands. Thankfully, with support from friends and family, I did not take his misguided advice.

An incident occurred at church a few years later that further challenged my faith. Rather than obey my pastor, who invoked scripture to insist I forgive a man who had endangered my child, I walked away from that church and from the power of misused scripture to control me. For years I wondered if I had any faith. And still, I attended church, a different church than I'd ever attended. It was an Episcopal church, related to C.S Lewis's Anglican Church, which Lewis referenced so often in his writing. This was my first encounter with formal liturgy, that is, recurring prayers used throughout the service, drawn from scripture and the oldest of church writings.

Church attendance was a life-long habit for me, yet felt deeply painful through that time. In the past I had always jumped into church life, eager to learn how I could give back, since I knew participation was a key to feeling part of a church community. In this time of pain, all I could take in was the music. Just let me sing the old hymns, I thought, the poetry of my childhood. Don't ask me to get otherwise involved.

It was as if the blinders were off. No longer could I embrace wholeheartedly the idea that any church was a safe place. Instead, I grappled with the knowledge that churches, and any community, are made of people who will disappoint. As difficult as it felt, these were important lessons I needed to learn. No community is without its difficulties.

Through these dark years, caring for my children and cleaning houses to pay our bills, a bright light appeared—the world of storytelling. It began the day I found myself agreeing to tell some stories to my daughter's kindergarten class. I had read stories to my son's class, but this slip of the tongue, to tell rather than read stories, plunged me into a world I had never known existed.

A friend pointed me in a direction to get me started. The goal was to set the book aside and simply telling a story. After my first visit as a storyteller, my daughter's teachers asked me to come back again, and yet again. Through this open door I discovered entirely different perspectives from what I had known, and met people from many walks of life, few of whom were overtly Christian, many not Christians at all. Yet I felt welcomed, loved, affirmed, and encouraged to keep learning and exploring how I could give back through the gifts I was developing. I told folk tales to different groups, and as I repeated the same stories to different audiences, the details of the tales changed subtly, perhaps even as I was changing. These stories played an important role in bringing about healing, compassion for myself, and forgiveness.

When in casual conversation with a fellow storyteller, I expressed my ambivalence about whether I was even a Christian. He laughed. "Give it up, Marjorie. You ARE a Christian." Well then. The "hound from heaven," a term used over the years to describe God's relentless pursuit of those he loves, was clearly not letting me go.

I felt sure this was the beginning of better times for me. I'd gained stable house-cleaning clients, a steady source of income that helped pay the majority of my bills. My storytelling performance schedule was lined up for months in advance,

The day I was felled by a seizure at age thirty-six marked a profound turning point. My ten-year-old daughter climbed over my seizing body to call our neighbor for help. A trip to the hospital quickly confirmed the existence of a massive meningioma—a brain tumor, the "good kind" that was less likely to kill me—that had to be removed.

Brain surgery is scary at the best of times. It was not clear I would survive. I said goodbye to my children before heading off to the hospital with my sister, unsure if I would ever see them again. In the car on the way to the hospital my sister, Beth, who had come to take me there, said, "It's OK to cry." I stared into an abyss.

I survived, only to wake from surgery to discover my entire right side was paralyzed. My life had been saved, yet I could not walk, get myself to the bathroom, roll over, or shift myself in bed. Working to support myself was out of the question; strongly right-handed, I had difficulty feeding myself with my left hand. How would I care for my children, much less myself? I felt totally dependent, frightened, and very angry.

Healing since that time has occurred in fits and starts and continues to this day. I am able to dance again, and walk on uneven trails with the support of my hiking poles. I drive limited distances after seven years off the road because of difficulty controlling my seizures. I've even written books about walking, guides along the theme of *Easy Walks,* for those who, like me, love nature and long to find places where they can feel safe in the outdoors. My solitude and inability to do other work drove me to learn to write, a skill I continue to polish as I write for local newspapers and do the work of helping families, including my own, to preserve their stories.

I've learned to live with and accommodate the limitations on my life. Keeping up with the pace of life in America is not something I will ever return to, and it turns out I don't miss the frenetic hurriedness that is part and parcel of that lifestyle. Instead, I use the quiet times to pray when I clean up from supper, while washing dishes, while ironing or preparing meals, or taking in the sunshine. As I've learned in further reading about monastic life, one's prayer and work are inextricably intertwined. The more mindless the work, the easier it is to pray.

My healthy grown children have given me grandgirls and grandboys who call me Grandma and love for me to read stories to them. I found love again after twenty years as a single parent, and Jon married me knowing the challenges I live with. He supports me in so many ways, including when we travel to see wonderful new places. He worked with a bike builder to make a tandem bicycle I can ride on, so I sit on the back and pedal while he provides the balance and strength for us to explore rail trails far and wide.

Church is a constant. When it's been too long since I've gotten to church, my husband is the one who says, "You need to go." He's right, so I do.

Surprise—2000

Sitting on the back of a horse named Surprise, I waited impatiently as the instructor adjusted the stirrups to fit my short legs. It was 1965, my first riding lesson at age nine. I was excited, and only a little anxious. Two instructors kept a close eye out as the class walked our horses around the ring. One of the instructors, wearing a raincoat against the damp, turned, the wind blowing open her coat. Frightened by the flashing fabric, my horse shied, nearly dislodging me from the saddle. Startled, I grabbed the saddle horn, dropping the reins.

Given free rein, my mount took off like a shot. The outer rail was temptingly close so I lunged, missed the railing, and ended up still on the horse, riding sideways. Holding on as my mount galloped about the ring, we provided a circus-like show for the enraptured students, who stood gaping at the spectacle. My frightened horse turned sharply, dumping me face first into a large mud puddle in the ring. Relieved of his frantic, noisy burden, he soon stopped. The instructors led him out of the ring, back to his stall.

Toweled off, I was placed right back on the most placid horse at the establishment and walked around the ring, the instructor holding the horse's head steady the entire outing. They knew the old adage, that the best thing to do when you fall off a horse is to get right back in the saddle.

Wary yet undeterred by my first outing, I continued taking lessons that year, and later rode at several other stables in the area. Throughout that time no other horse offered a ride that came close to my first misadventure. I developed a taste for gentle cantering, much preferring the rolling gait to the bumpity-bump of trotting, with its attendant jouncing of the spine. And much nicer than the terrifying feeling of being on board a runaway.

As an adult, my enthusiasm for horseback riding was always attended by trepidation. I longed to glide along on the back of a quiet horse. There was always the possibility, especially with an unfamiliar horse, that her plans and mine would not coincide. I thought my discomfort must be because I'd never had much occasion to care for a horse. Maybe the mucking out, feeding, saddling, and general handling of the animal might have lessened my anxiety. In truth, my enthusiasm was always compromised by the suspicion that something untoward was likely to happen.

My health issues later made horseback riding and even walking more difficult for me. While I had enjoyed the sensation of being on the back of a horse, I didn't miss the anxiety of coping with a large animal.

One weekend with my extended family, we gathered to remember my mother, who had died earlier that year. We stayed with Mom's oldest and dearest friends, Audrey and Alan, at their lakeside cottage in Maine. While there, I spotted some small, sit-on-top kayaks. My children, their cousins, and my siblings, took the kayaks out on the quiet lake, paddling and maneuvering with ease on the surface of the water. Unlike river kayaks, these small recreational kayaks are stable and easy to steer, intended for quiet paddles in calm waters, not dashing through white-water rapids. Despite my mobility issues, I felt compelled to try one of the little boats. They looked just my speed.

Getting help to climb onto one of the kayaks, I pushed off and was entranced. I flashed back to my experiences riding on horseback. When a passing boat sent a rolling wake my direction, I rode the swells, which brought to mind the sensation of a horse's gentle cantering gait. It was both comforting and reassuring. I hated returning to shore. This was a way for me to move with grace again, something I had been deprived of for many years. After taking short breaks I'd head back out, getting in a last paddle the morning we left.

Once back home at Silver Lake, I kept thinking of that small kayak and the pleasure I'd had paddling. As a disabled single parent, my finances did not allow for the purchase of a kayak. My siblings saw my joy and soon my sister Beth arrived at my house with a joint gift from them: a little red kayak. We took it out on Silver Lake to christen it. Since then my small boat has traveled many miles with me.

On one of our first dates, my second husband and I paddled our kayaks on the river near where he lived. There we confirmed our mutual joy in nature, and our shared passion of being on the water in our little watercraft. Floating along the river, we passed others paddling their kayaks and canoes. We spoke together with ease as we followed the course of the river, playfully bumping each other's boats as we wandered from shore to shore, exploring the river.

The great blue herons played hide and seek among the grasses, flying just ahead of us, then settling down, squawking as we came up beside them farther along the river. Shy turtles nosedived into the water, disappearing from sight.

These days we still to paddle quiet waterways. We added a tandem kayak to our small flotilla, a sleek vessel that steers easily. Our paddles knife through the water in rhythm as we move through the water in silence.

The day I settled into the seat of that little kayak in Maine, I was surprised in a much different way than on my first encounter with a horse in the riding ring. The first strokes of my paddle moved the boat through the water with ease. There were similarities to my horseback riding experiences, but I was grateful for the differences. Evidently I had been searching for a little boat to love all that time.

When I am paddling, my heart sings. When life feels hard, my kayak offers a refuge, a comfort, until I'm ready to face the day. Alone or with companions, I'm filled with joy as I glide along.

Everyone needs a "little boat" in their life. How lucky for me that mine is waiting at the lake, and as far as I know, has never even thought of running away with me.

Keep on Singing—1999

First published in Alive Now! Upper Room Ministries, 2010,
reprinted with permission

I was part of the choir that was preparing to perform some "greatest hits" from Handel's *Messiah*. As I sat through the dress rehearsal, I had my doubts if everything would come together. The director stopped us in so many places, focusing on tone, pitch, pronunciation, articulation. I felt like I was in a car with someone just learning to drive as we jerked down the road. I wanted to say, "Clutch—put in the clutch!" It was a bumpy ride.

During the rehearsal, in which most of the soloists practiced their parts with us so we could get a feel for how those parts fit into the program, the director made an important point. A soloist had made an error of omission, leaving out a few words in the solo. He instructed us, the choir, to resist following along in the musical score when the soloists were singing. "If you do this and see a mistake," he explained, "you won't be able to help reacting, which will draw attention to it. The audience will see your reaction. Just sit back and enjoy the music. I will cue you to when to come back in."

He was firm on this point: "No looking!" What I didn't realize until after the performance to a standing-room-only crowd was that during the performance all the nitpicking that he had done during the rehearsal was also done. Were there mistakes? Oh, yes. Did he stop and correct us? Not once. He gave no indication that we had made mistakes.

We just kept singing. When the last notes were sung, the crowd greeted us with loud, appreciative applause. They had not come hoping to pick out mistakes. Nor did they come expecting perfection, or novelty. They found joy in the familiar, and comfort in the majestic sounds of Handel's music.

Each of us will find good reasons to focus on mistakes, while other times we must just "keep singing." May we have the wisdom to recognize the difference and respond accordingly.

Responsible Worrying—1998

My friend and I were visiting together. Our conversation rambled, straying to topics we wanted to bounce off someone we knew would listen without providing a ready answer. We are both pretty grounded and capable of figuring out a lot on our own. It's the "being listened to" that is important, not the providing of solutions.

We came to the topic of friends who appeared to have intractable problems, and how sad we feel when we know there is no way we can fix their problem. When I was going through some of my hardest struggles, this friend was able to listen to me even though she could do little to put things right. Perhaps more important than the listening, I knew that she cared, yet didn't allow her caring to destroy her own love of life, her enjoyment of her children, and her joy in the outdoors. Because she was taking care of herself, I was able to talk about my struggles and know she would "worry responsibly." I felt confident that it would not be too hard for her. She didn't let my problems destroy her joy.

As I have grown stronger and am more able to carry others' burdens for a time, it is easier to be a "responsible worrier." To care deeply, and then allow myself to go dancing, and let my body, heart, and soul fly as freely as the music can carry me. To laugh or weep with my friends and then return to the presence of my children, who often make me laugh till tears roll down my cheeks.

We are thinking of issuing "Responsible Worrier" cards, whose membership requires "Deep caring, intent listening, respect of personal privacy, and a determination to do what is needful if it is possible. To speak to someone who is able to help if possible, to promise to pray, even when there seems no clear solution. To trust God to care as much as we do (well, maybe God can care more ...) as we rejoice in the gifts we are given. And when we are called to 'worry responsibly' again, we will have the strength and the will to do so with a grateful heart."

I think this must be an organization that is self-selected. If we had to decide who could and could not join, it would just be another thing to worry about.

Grace in Unexpected Places—2000

I saw my divorce lawyer recently. It had been awhile. He greeted me and introduced me to his wife. I told them what a compassionate divorce lawyer he was. He responded, "That's an enigma, isn't it?" We all laughed.

I never dreamed I would need a divorce lawyer. It was 1985 and I had been married for ten years. I was in no shape, emotionally or physically, to look around for the "very best." I called him because he was "a friend of a friend," and went from there.

Contrary to stereotypes, from the beginning of my dealings with him he guided me towards a possible solution, not an impossible ideal. For my first appearance in court, he drove with me, explained what to expect, and sat by my side as we negotiated child support arrangements. My world had turned upside down.

As we drove back home, rather than discuss further strategy, what else I could have said, or anything of that sort, he told me stories. Stories of his own family, some of their dealings, disagreements, and how they had solved some of their problems. He spoke of both his and his wife's pride in their children. How, beyond either of their professional accomplishments, the warmth they felt towards their children far surpassed any pride they experienced from their own work.

I had little to say then. I think he knew, or sensed that I was in a place of deep despair. He didn't look for any response, instead filled the time we spent together offering a caring warmth that comforted me as much as was possible at the time. I have never forgotten that. We have had a few dealings since that first terrifying trip to court so many years ago but none were as hard as the first.

I hear the lawyer jokes, but never having been much of a joke teller myself, I have not passed them on. In fact, I don't have much enthusiasm for jokes, especially not lawyer jokes. When I needed an advocate, one who had the strength to speak for me when I felt too downtrodden to speak for myself, I found someone who spoke for me. Rather than pointing out what I should have done, how I "should" have advocated for myself, he told me stories. When there was no spirit in me to do what needed to be done, a compassionate lawyer stayed near me and stood up for me and my children. An enigma? I call it a gift.

There's Hope—2000

I have felt close to some neighbors. We've shared meals, taken walks together, traded kid-watching responsibilities, and loaned one another eggs, butter, or sugar. Others have remained in the acquaintance category. They always smile, I smile back, yet we had never tried to have a conversation.

Half-way through one summer, I heard that a neighbor's young son had died. Though I hadn't known the parents, I had known this "child," for a child is how I still thought of him, even though he was in his twenties by then, not much older than my oldest. We had spent long waits together at the bus stop. After high school he had moved away from home, and it had been several months since he had died. No one in the neighborhood seemed to have known about it.

Once I heard the news I looked for a good time to say something to the mother. I felt awkward going to the door and announcing that I was paying a condolence call several months late, when we had never exchanged visits before.

One morning I strolled down the hill in the bright sunshine, spring in the air. She was in her back yard, rake in hand, cleaning up. I said, "Hello." She threw her head back and cried out, "There's hope!" We laughed. I agreed that spring was on its way, then went on my way.

I haven't been able to get her words out of my head. She, who had lost her only son, was able to look at the world around her and pronounce, "There's hope!" and then laughed with me. I didn't feel a lack of words, so much as a humbling of spirit.

She and I have met up with each other many times since, and often speak from the heart. It turned out we have plenty to say to each other. Had she changed, or had I? It doesn't really matter. What is important is that we found a way to bridge the gap and speak of her son with love. I know she has not forgotten, and she seems to find some comfort from the fact that I remember too.

Climbing Mountains—2010

I sat in the pew, surrounded by a grieving family. They were distraught. The deceased—their beloved mother and grandmother—had died after struggling with cancer for several years.

The priest was reflecting on the Gospel reading, the end of which included the Sermon on the Mount. That's when he talked about a bit of wisdom he'd acquired in his seminary days: "If you head to the top of a mountain, something important is going to happen."

Although I sat in church, many miles from any mountains, my thoughts wandered. The priest's words reminded me of a time that I had reached the summit of two mountains at Acadia National Park, one by car and the other on foot.

We used the car to get me up Cadillac Mountain, where we had a 360 degree view encompassing Frenchman Bay and the Atlantic Ocean. Our walk up the carriage road to the top of Day Mountain was slow. We found lots of plants and rocks to examine on the way. The higher we climbed, the better the view of the ocean and numerous islands just off-shore. It was early June, and the cranberry plants were in full flower. We stopped often to enjoy the pinkish hues of the cranberry flowers along the carriage path we followed as it wound around the mountain. Occasional lady slippers revealed themselves as we climbed.

Chattering fellow travelers disturbed the quiet. Didn't they notice the stillness? We slowed as though to study the cranberries more closely, allowing the talkative walkers to pass. Soon, we again climbed alone in silence. We found at the summit a lumpy plateau, with plenty of great spots where we could sit and take in the views. We settled in and looked out toward the ocean.

We headed back down since the weather was changing. The wind began to blow and dark clouds rolled in. I hoped we could get down before we were caught in a downpour.

Once we came down off the mountain, a swamp lay in front of us. The trail we needed to follow was made of long narrow planks offering great footing for some, but not for me. As though on a balance beam, I wobbled as my husband spotted me, offering a hand as he traipsed beside me through the muck. I was relieved to emerge from the swamp without having tumbled into the mud myself.

We went one last time to Cadillac Mountain before leaving for home the next morning. It was a clear sky, so we drove to the top and waited for the sun to go down. As it grew dark stars began to appear. We found a relatively flat rock to lie down on and looked skyward.

I searched in vain for Orion's belt; it must have been tucked in a different part of the sky. The big dipper looked ready to pour out its contents into the night sky. And then, off to the left, a shooting star flashed past—joy!

I have often spent time staring up into the night sky only to hear from a companion, "A shooting star!" which had already disappeared when I turned my head. Holding my head still and waiting, this time I was the one who saw the star racing through the night.

Leaving those thoughts aside, my attention returned to the grieving family that surrounded me. They were climbing a different mountain than I had been thinking of, the mountain of grief. I could not do that work for them. What I could do was let them know they were not alone. When climbing a mountain, you're likely to find something different than you anticipated. First, however, you must start, however you can.

Sacred Housecleaning—2008

Near the end of the church service that day, I watched our priest finish serving the Eucharist. It is a ritualized process each week, almost a dance, with each person at the altar doing their part.

For those of us in the pews, our experiences vary. Wiggly children next to or behind us attract our attention. Friends exchange smiles. Some take time for quiet reflection that can be claimed even in a full church.

I was struck by a different perspective as our priest walked through his ritualized cleanup routine that follows after each serving of the Eucharist. Bread and wine, the vessels he used to serve them, and others to clean, were all at hand. He ate the leftover wafers, as is the custom in the Anglican tradition, drank the leftover wine, then waited for the acolyte to hand him the vial of water to rinse the small glass pitcher that had held the wine. After wiping the second cup clean, he placed it on the altar, then covered all with a cloth.

It was then that I grasped the sanctity of this work. Our priest was performing a housecleaning chore. Clearing up after a meal, carefully, with reverence, respect, and knowledge of the sacred. With an entire congregation for his audience to boot! Recognizing this I felt stunned. In front of me was a model of the sacredness of tasks we face each day; to feed and care for our families, and to clean up and prepare for the next meal, with gratitude, acknowledging that there will be a "next time."

As we sat, ostensibly the audience for this ceremony, our attention was elsewhere—children, friends, our own thoughts or prayers. How like normal life. We often toil alone in our daily tasks, unnoticed, and rarely appreciated.

This made our priest's work even more poignant; he was doing the work of serving, feeding and cleaning, unnoticed and perhaps not even recognized, much as the rest of us go about the daily chores that are required to keep our families going. Physical necessities are often noticed only when absent, rarely commented on when attended to each day. This, however, does not eliminate the sacredness of the task.

It is hard to remain focused and to persist in our efforts when our work is undone or ignored. The difficulty is part of what makes it important. Little that is sacred in life is easy, even if we wish it were so.

Zen Dishes—2010

I returned to my home life after surgery and initial rehabilitation in 1993 weakened, yet desperate to do anything. When I had been at the rehab hospital the staff had insisted we inmates (patients, that is) perform what they called "standing therapy." We were encouraged, teased, and cajoled into standing for periods of fifteen minutes at a time. Most of those in rehab with me were stroke victims, almost all elderly, and they needed a lot of cajoling. I was much younger than the others, needed no cajoling, and resented the undisguised condescension in the therapists' voices.

We stood around a table in groups of four or five, an aide standing nearby in case any of us keeled over or decided to sit down prematurely, as we played card games or games of block-stacking. Mostly these activities consisted of "Concentration," something I was never good at and especially not then.

Once I returned home, we developed what became a running family joke, pointing out all the things I did that were "standing therapy." Making my bed, lifting open windows to the fresh spring air, and hanging out clothes on the clothes line were part of my rehabilitation. Each clothes pin I squeezed when hanging out clothes on the line helped my fingers to grow stronger.

These tasks were helpful in restoring function, but washing dishes became my favorite therapy. The warm, soapy water soothed my aching right arm and shoulder as I worked to reawaken and strengthen muscles that had been paralyzed and were beginning to regain function. The view at my sink as I worked was (and still is) out my kitchen window, where neighborhood children, including my own, played on the swings or ran about in the yard. The woods at the edge of our yard that spring had begun greening up.

The choice of dishes we used for meals became a point of grace. We decided as a family to put away the heavy earthenware dinner plates we had always used, pulling out our much lighter Corelle™ plates. The difference in weight allowed me to enjoy the after dinner cleanup in the warm, soapy water before the pain in my shoulder became too severe. Each session at the sink after a meal was a sweet reminder of small yet loving choices my family made for my sake. The real joy was that I had the liberty to stop as soon as it hurt, which varied according to what else I had attempted to do that day.

My parents stayed with us for several months after my surgery. A family member, either a child or grandparent, was always ready and usually cheerful to step in when I put the dishcloth down. Trying to push through, or rushing to finish the dishes myself, taught me another important lesson in healing: Trying harder doesn't always work. When the pain in my shoulder became too much to bear, I had to stop and allow healing to progress at its own pace.

And so, Zen Dishes. As I stood at the soap-filled sink, family members often wandered by. They were not interfering, just checking to make sure I was all right. I usually declined an offer of help with the explanation, "No, it feels so good to do this. Please don't make me stop." Thus, our family developed the tongue-in-cheek joke, "Don't bother Mom, she's doing her Zen dishes." And I was.

157

I still enjoy doing dishes, although I am much more willing these days to be gracious when help is offered. The thing about Zen is that it goes where you are. My life, by God's gracious gift, has moved beyond doing dishes. If I had not had that time to heal, this might have been a very different story.

Seeing in the Dark—1999

It was dark when we arrived that Friday night in Rockport, Massachusetts. We planned to attend a wedding the next day and had been offered a place overlooking the ocean where we could spend the night. The owner had advised us to bring our own flashlights, a puzzling warning. We arrived and had trouble finding the apartment unit, since it lacked any porch lighting. Once we turned our flashlights on we saw that yes, it was right where the owner had told us it would be.

My sister Mary Glen had driven out from Boston to pick us up and drive with us to Rockport: she was also attending the wedding. As my daughter and I went about our usual cross-purposes when faced with a new environment (me: check out all the details, figure out the necessities, she: explore all the neat corners and figure out all the gadgets and buttons and exactly how all of them work) my sister stayed the strong middle course and pointed out sensible solutions to problems I found overwhelming. We managed well considering our differing personalities.

I finally settled into bed with a book to wind down before sleep. After reading a chapter in the book I brought, I reached over to switch off the lamp. No sooner than I had rested my head on the pillow I sat right back up, stunned by what was out my window.

I knew we were at the ocean. We had driven past the shoreline as we turned into the condo area. I had seen pictures of the beach and the rocks along the shoreline. Caught up in the details of getting settled, the necessary decisions and the practical ones, I missed what was right in front of me. It was as if I was blind. In fact, as long as the lights were on, I couldn't see out if I'd tried.

In the darkest of night, I was finally able to take in what was there. Glittering lights in the tiny inlet across the way twinkled and sparkled against the water's surface. It had been waiting for me all along. The lights of Rockport reflected on the incoming waves as they headed to the shore. The sea was calm, with little wind. With the windows closed, I had been unable to hear the waves wash onto the sand. In silent witness of the quiet rhythms of the ocean, I was finally able to see.

Finding Easy Walks—2020

Many woodland paths at Acadia National Park, a place we visit often, are filled with roots and rocks. On our outings there we sometimes encounter walkways created from narrow boards or find trails near steep drop-offs. These present the risk of serious injury for me. Searching out easier places for me where I can relax and enjoy my surroundings has become a family quest.

In the last few years this has expanded far beyond Acadia and has continued in our outings near home and across the U.S. When we have been able, we have visited beyond its borders into Canada and Ireland, finding Easy Walks in these far-flung locations.

Our family has codified this into the phrase, Easy Walks, the name I gave to my hiking book series. The first three books focus on trails near our home in Massachusetts. When my husband and I travel farther afield, we seek out the same types of trails that offer me the freedom to move safely, which has given me the experience to write yet another book, *Finding Easy Walks Wherever You Are.*

As I became more adept at navigating paths independently, it felt frustrating hearing about trails I could not enjoy. Rail trails have been and are being developed, both locally and farther from home, with water views, overlooks, and a chance to enjoy wildlife along the way. I wanted to explore them, and my feet could not get me there.

We searched for a tandem bicycle with no cross bar, so I could get on it. I needed pedals in a foot forward position to help; Pedals I could keep my foot on were essential. We discovered a style of bike that met these requirements and obtained one. The outdoor world opened up for me.

We set out for a bike ride along the carriage trails of Acadia National Park on a day that was growing quite warm. We had lots of cooling gear with us and stopped in shady spots. My husband monitored me to ensure that I was not getting hot, and we stopped frequently to spray me down, keep me cool. We went up and down the hilly carriage trails. I am able to provide some assistance in the pedaling, yet most of the burden is on Jon to propel us forward.

We were reminded of one of the most important aspects of accepting assistance: being sure our support staff arc not burned out. Those who offer support need the freedom to take breaks and renew their own energies. After our difficult pedal along the carriage trails of the park, we made sure Jon got out for a hike alone.

He set out on a challenging trail that promised views of the ocean, and enjoyed some rock hopping along the shore. None of that was inviting for me. It was just what he needed.

My husband has walked with me on many of the trails that are included in my *Easy Walks* books. I have also explored many areas accompanied by a host of other willing walkers. Friends and family members are not always familiar with my health concerns. When I let them know my needs, they have been great listeners, compassionate, kind, and ready to offer a hand. I have worked hard to learn to communicate how they can help keep me safe. It's a life lesson I get to practice often.

Easy Walks are not just about enjoying time in nature. My book series has become a way to share this passion with others. Through this work I have made new friends. Discovering tools that have eased my path has been a source of healing.

My limits continue to change. It is hard when I hit these boundaries. Despite my frustrations, I still look forward to time spent outside with others. That is a gift I feel grateful for every day.

Life is Messy—1998

In the early days of watching my marriage dissolve I came across a book that suggested housecleaning as a viable way to support oneself. Seizing on this idea, I found a friend who took me in hand and taught me the basics. She invited me to clean her house for pay, then offered a reference so I could obtain other business. With little money and few ideas for how I was to care for my children, housecleaning became an unexpected gift that helped me support our family until I became ill seven years later.

It was 1987 and my children were young. My kids were home from school. With no place to leave them, I brought them with me to the house I was cleaning. I worked and tried to make sure my kids were not undoing what I had done. They were good, just bored.

My daughter discovered a set of finger paints on the family's toy shelf, and announced she wanted to do some finger painting. I rarely had the nerve to suggest finger painting in my own house. Life felt messy enough without inviting yet more disarray into our home.

I explained that I was there to clean up this house, not create more messes. She nodded and slid the finger paints back onto the shelf where she'd found them. Dropping down on the floor next to her brother, they sat in front of the television and let me finish my work

Feeling sad about denying her this simple, yet problematic request, a thought intruded: Life is messy, birth is messy, death is messy. If there's life, it's going to be messy. If it's not messy, it's not life. It felt like a cosmic joke that I found housecleaning to be so satisfying when my own life, my own house, felt so topsy-turvy.

No, I didn't change my mind and set up finger paints for my little girl at my client's house. Having had an insight I have pondered countless times since did not make embracing mess any easier.

I have recalled these words often, particularly when I hear others complain about the terrible state of (fill in your blank). I try to remind them, "Life is messy. Birth is messy. Death is messy. Why in the world should what happens in between those times be different? If it were, it wouldn't be life. It might be something else, but not life." Each time I speak these words, I am speaking first and foremost to myself.

Solitude—1998

In ninth-grade English, I got a homework assignment to make up a collage of pictures conveying the idea of solitude. Collages were a common project in my junior high-high school years. They typically consisted of magazine photos slapped onto poster board in a wild array. I had little material to work with. My classmates brought in collages featuring celebrities, flashy jewelry, and sun-swept beaches. Our family subscribed to no magazines that featured such graphics.

We had a few magazines, and I found some "quiet" pictures: a small boy climbing on a fallen tree trunk, and a plane soaring across a vast horizon. To me, these were images conveyed peace, stillness, quiet. I arranged them on a poster board, filling the space with solitude, serenity, quiet, and structure. My teacher stared at my finished piece, bewildered.

"What is this?" she asked. I explained that it represented how solitude felt to me. "Oh," she countered. "When I'm home alone, I want to take my shoes off, kick back, and make a mess if I want. That's what solitude is to me." I suspected she was disappointed there was no crazy array of images, as others in my class had created.

I responded, "That's not what it is to me at all." I sensed that here was a grown-up who had little grasped on something I had already discovered to be a precious gem—the joy, reverence, and sanctity of quiet. No TVs, no party atmosphere, no radios, only peace, stillness, and silence.

The image of the small boy climbing the length of a fallen tree trunk has stayed with me, among all the photos I included for that project. I knew that many small children understand solitude, reverence, and respect for sanctuary. It feels like ancient wisdom that is easy to forget as we grow older.

Even in her lack of understanding, this teacher was able to give me a gift. It may be how we receive more than we know.

Spectator or Participant—2015

First published in "True Stories Well Told," website. June 15, 2015

Many of my early school years were spent as a spectator. I was always the one to wait, and to let others go first. I wanted to see what might happen before I tiptoed into a new experience.

In my last year of high school I felt restless. When my friends told me the swim team needed an additional springboard diver to constitute a team for competition, with their encouragement, I "dove" in.

I have an aversion to heights—something happens in my gut when I peer over the edge of a seeming abyss. Here I was standing on the edge of a diving board, being asking to increase my distance from the water. When I first stood at the end of the 1-meter diving board and was urged, "Jump up," all I wanted to do was to get down as fast as possible.

That's where Mr. Crane came in. The parent of one of my fellow divers, he arrived after work each afternoon in his coat and tie, ready to watch and advise us in our diving efforts. As soon as he stood at the edge of the pool we began taking our turns on the board in earnest.

Among us were two state diving champions, another who came in close to top in the state, a few experienced divers, and me. It didn't matter—we each got his undivided attention, precise suggestions, and his encouragement to try again.

For an entire year, I headed to the pool each day after school, wriggled into my bathing suit, and hit the water. Learning each new dive felt terrifying, and six different "dives" were required to compete. Mr. Crane metaphorically held my hand as I struggled to learn each of the main dives: back dive, front dive, inward, reverse, half twist, and forward 1½. By the end of the year, I had made it. I could complete these six dives, more or less, with some degree of skill.

One day another coach approached me, asking if I would like to add a few more dives to my list so I could help the team participate in a larger event. "Uh, no, I don't think so," was my answer. I'd reached the limit of my short-lived springboard diving career.

When I left for college, people wondered if I would continue to dive. Not a chance. College diving starts with the 3-meter board and moves on up to the 10-meter platform—thirty feet up. This was not my cup of tea at all. But I had learned that I could step out of the crowd, stop being a spectator, and participate.

I later learned that Mr. Crane had never been on a diving board in his life. I had no idea whether he could even swim. It didn't matter. He paid attention, understood how bodies moved, and was able to teach us. Whether he could dive or not was immaterial. He stood at the pool's edge in his coat, tie, and business trousers, and described what we each needed to do to be more skillful, and better able to cut a clean line into the water as we dove. And it worked.

I have often looked back on this time, and felt such deep gratitude, not only for those friends who encouraged me to try, but for

Mr. Crane, who offered me his attention, regardless of what I might do with it. He was my model for what teaching is about—showing up, being there, offering encouragement, and not worrying about the end result. I have carried these experiences with me throughout many different life circumstances.

Another lesson learned? That, like Mr. Crane, I didn't always have to go out on a limb or a diving board to be able to help others. With my feet planted on the ground I can let my eyes, my voice, and my heart travel wherever others need me.

Telling Stories—2001

I was sure they would all stand up and walk out on me. Convinced of this, I had stayed away from working with groups of children. Then my own were born, drawing me into the world of working with little ones. I learned that the gentle approach—inviting rather than demanding—produced surprising results. Sometimes.

A slip of the tongue, as it seemed, brought me to the front of my daughter's kindergarten class that day in 1988. I had meant to say that I would read some stories to her class, as I had done for my son's classes the previous several years. Somehow the word "tell" rather than "read" came out, and once said, there was no backing down.

An acquaintance who was a professional storyteller recommended I use a particular tale that included a recurring brief song. The singing was important and gave the children a chance to participate in the story. As I grasped the structure for involving children in my presentation, I included an additional folk tale to fill out my time with them.

I got out my dusty guitar and practiced a few chords I had learned back in high school. My children and I had spent countless hours singing children's songs together so I included some of those tunes during the hour I spent with the children. I soon found myself in front of fifty eager kindergarteners and jumped in.

I solicited their help in creating new verses to the children's songs I taught them, and the time flew by. They chimed in on the repetitive phrases I taught them in the each story.

Afterwards the teachers greeted me with, "Can you come back next month?"

"Sure," I responded, realizing I'd have to come up with some new material. Hearing about a local storytelling festival, I made my way there. I soon learned new stories to use with these kindergarteners the following month, and the month after that.

My own children helped by being receptive story listeners, sitting with me as I combed through collections of folk tales. We discovered gems in dusty old books I found at used bookstores. "This would be a good story for you," my daughter often suggested.

When I heard that a small school nearby needed a music teacher, I approached them with the suggestion that they might really need a music and storytelling teacher. At the end of the interview, we agreed to give it a try.

For the next nine years, I had a consistent group of kids to practice new stories on. I pulled together songs, stories, and dances that kept kindergarteners through sixth graders moving, singing, and creating stories with me. They became my experimental lab in which new tales were tested out. They began to ask if that day's story would be told to other children. They had learned that I wanted their feedback. They were brutally honest.

As I took on paid performances, I gained confidence, believing I had gifts to give. Over the next fifteen years, the world of professional storytelling opened many doors for me. Storytellers and musicians became my friends and were generous with their time and experience. We related both our successes and failures. Always ready to offer suggestions, or lend an ear, they expressed confidence in my abilities and encouraged me to attempt things I had never dreamed possible.

Some of the secrets I learned? As much as you can, include everyone. State your expectations up front. If you're introducing something children are likely to be unfamiliar with, explain it briefly, with not too much detail. Walk them through what is coming, before beginning in earnest.

I also learned that music entices, invites, and urges children to move. Make space for them to respond. Act confident, even if you don't feel it, and never lash out—it achieves nothing.

Humor, humor, humor. Be willing to look silly, and never ridicule. Respect, respect, respect. Believe that your audience wants you to succeed, and never apologize. As much as possible, structure your time so the children feel they are in control. Convey your faith in them. And if things start getting out of control, whisper. Children just can't resist the possibility that they're missing something. Grownups have been known to feel this way too.

Finding a Way Back—2016

I have heard it said that understanding and sharing your past can change your future, yet it was years before I fully grasped this truth. In my work as a freelance writer and personal historian, I have often asked, "How did you get to where you are today?" The question might be about a person's vocation, or how they came to live in a certain place, or any other life situation that was worth reflecting upon. The answers I've gotten have been fascinating.

One day I asked the question of myself. I'd been invited to speak to a local Chamber of Commerce. They asked if I would talk about some history of the town where I had been asked to speak. "Sure," I answered. And then scrambled to figure out what I would say.

I soon realized that I knew quite a lot about the town of Walpole, Massachusetts. I began my talk by suggesting that I'd get different answers from each person, if I asked them how they'd come to Walpole.

"So how did a Florida girl end up here?" I asked. "I came north for college—and snow!"

I got what I wished for and have seen snow many times since. Coming to Walpole though? "What brought me to Walpole was love. You see … there was a boy."

Walpole is known to many only as a Massachusetts town that has a maximum security state prison. The town has other more positive features. I recalled the days when this young man who first brought me to Walpole. He worked for a local company, makers of cedar fences and buildings. People had been coming to Walpole since colonial days cut rot-resistant wood from its cedar swamp. Remnants of the swamp remain along the road from Walpole to the neighboring towns of Norfolk and Wrentham.

I was married at a tiny church tucked into the edge of Bird Park, a gift to the town from the wealthy Bird family. Members of the Chamber of Commerce audience smiled as I recalled the town swimming pool that had been built out of a small dammed stream in park. The waters of that stream eventually flow into the nearby Neponset River. By the time I came to Walpole, the pool had been abandoned in favor of a modern concrete town pool built in the downtown area.

Bird Park fell on hard times. It was not just because of the abandoned swimming pool. The wooded trails of the park were the scene of a grisly murder. People avoided the park, which made things worse.

It was not only Bird Park that fell on hard times. The marriage I had entered into with such hope fell on hard times too, ending in divorce. For many years afterwards I avoided Walpole, feeling reluctant to revisit places that had brought me joy, but afterwards brought such painful memories.

A few years ago, living in a nearby town, I began searching out local walking trails to create my first hiking book, *Easy Walks in Massachusetts*. As the book series expanded and I traveled to other nearby towns, walking and documenting local trails, I got closer and closer to Walpole. What I found when I returned was not what I had remembered.

Bird Park had been taken over by the Trustees of Reservations and transformed into a little jewel of open space. It had become a place where families could once more enjoy time together. The swimming pool had been restored to a more natural state. I brought my grandgirl to the park and watched as she stared, eye to eye, with a large bullfrog hunkered down in the weeds of what had become the frog pond.

The Walpole Town Forest offered some of the best views in the area of the Upper Neponset River. Adams Farm, a very recent addition to town open space, was a wonderful gift to the town, with trails and a community garden.

I ended with a story I had heard of an adopted son who felt like he didn't belong. His family undertook a DNA genealogy study, the results of which revealed that many generations back, forbears of that adopted son had been connected to his adoptive family. In joining this family, a long-lost son had returned home.

It was a simple question I had been asked. "Can you share any Walpole history?" My answer was more complicated. After my talk, men and women huddled together in conversation, their memories spurred by stories I had told. This Florida girl had felt like an outsider ever since she came to New England. The day I spoke with the generous folks in Walpole, I felt as if I'd come home. Sharing our past may change our future. And that's a very good thing.

Learning to Swim—2010

It's not surprising that because I grew up in Florida, some of my earliest memories have to do with water. The heat, the ubiquity of swimming pools, the ocean, and the hot weather make it a consistent presence in this near-tropical part of the country.

There is a difference between "swimming" and "paddling about." The latter is something that small, and not so small, children can do in the shallows of calm beaches. The former requires being able to let go of the security of touching the bottom of the pool or the sand beneath one's feet. As a child I did quite a lot of paddling and not much swimming.

A near-drowning incident in which I stepped into a water-filled hole created by a broken fire hydrant made me wary. Despite this fright, I still liked cool, wet places, as long as it wasn't a muddy puddle of unknown depth.

At neighbor's pools and in the ocean, I whirled my hands as it appeared my siblings, cousins and other relatives did. Without fail I sank like a stone, albeit a splashing stone.

After another failed attempt to swim like my siblings and cousins, my Aunt Betty took me aside from the crowd and spoke to me in a quiet voice, as was her habit. She had watched what I was doing and offered a suggestion. Holding her hands up in front of her, she said, "Take your hands and cup them like so." Demonstrating by squeezing her fingers together, then bending them to make small scoops, she pulled her hand through the water. "Then move through the water like this," and she reached out and slowly drew her arm past her, creating a small wake as she demonstrated.

A light bulb went on in my five year old head. Her quiet manner, her gentle way of speaking, and her belief in me allowed me to believe that I could do what she had showed me. "Now put your face down and pull hard!"

I took a deep breath, pushed off and concentrated on pulling the water past me, rather than fighting against it. I soon felt myself floating near the surface. As I moved, I was buoyed up, rather than sinking. I could swim!

While I recall nothing after that moment, I suspect my family found it difficult to get out of the water that day. I began to experiment, discovering that steady kicking gave my arms an additional assist as I moved. Swimming underwater was even easier, since used great sweeping motions with my arms and legs to glide under the surface.

I soon came to love opening my eyes in the saltwater that was right in front of my grandmother's beach house. My cousins and I played games together, looking for hidden objects on the sandy bottom.

Although I could now swim, I longed to float, something my mother and grandmother did with ease as they bobbed on the surface like corks, their toes popping up as they leisurely rested their arms behind their heads. My efforts produced only a slow sinking experience, my feet dragging the rest of me down to the sandy bottom.

I tried all the tricks offered, holding my breath, stretching my arms way behind my head; but none of them worked. I resigned myself to waving my hands alongside my legs, back and forth, palms down, a motion called "sculling." It always felt like cheating to me.

I took a class in high school to become a swimming teacher. The rigorous training helped me realize that I could show others how to float quite well—I already knew all the tricks. What I had to be careful of when demonstrating was not to do it for too long; I would then be exposed as a sinker.

Both children and adults learned to float as I worked with them. Some, however, were just not going to float on their backs, regardless of their best efforts. I was able to console them. "Float on your stomach—it's called survival floating," I'd then say. "You can still try on your back, but here's what you'll need to do to keep your head above water." I'd show them the simple sculling motion I'd learned so long before. It worked.

Some aspects of swimming came to me in a flash, the light bulb experience that is so exciting when it happens. I acquired other skills through experimentation, observation, adaptation, and practice. If I hadn't had that first flash of understanding I might not have persisted in my efforts. My aunt has always downplayed her part in the process. I assure her, "It may not have been much, but it was what I needed and made all the difference"

Did I Tell You This?—2000

I received an essay from a friend beset by Parkinson's, the gist of which was that he was worried about repeating himself, telling the same story over again. This is how I answered him:

Dear Bob, rather than always listening to the details of a story, it helps to pay attention to why a person is sharing the story—again. I have retold countless times about the day I learned to swim—that eureka! moment when my aunt suggested I cup my hands, and suddenly I was able to do what up that point had been unattainable.

With each retelling, I find myself reframing it, recognizing that it has been something I've talked about many times. Yet each retelling reflects changes in my own life, perspectives, growth, and even self-forgiveness. It may also reveal related experiences of healing. Many of these lessons were learned not because of trying harder, but because the time was right and my body was ready.

There is great value in stories we repeat. In fact, children love to be read the same books over and over and find both reassurance and comfort in the familiar. When young, my children would request, when someone is visiting, that I retell a story that cast them in a funny light—that focused the attention on them. We all laughed, knowing how it came out (minus the new listener), and at the end of the story this person was drawn into our family lore.

Yes, I do worry about repeating myself in writing. However, just as we gain a different perspective when rereading a favorite book, perhaps our listeners will take something different or new from our stories, even as we learn something ourselves in the retelling. The tales may have changed from the last time, since it is possible we've lived and learned as time has passed.

The Tears Won't Come—2020

After taking the classes required to teach swimming lessons, I spent several summers as a swimming instructor at a local pool. Walking toward me one day was a sullen little girl with her grandparents. Her hair was unbrushed, and it was obvious that she wished to be somewhere, anywhere else than where she found herself. Her body language all but screamed, "Get me out of here!" as she stood on the pool deck, eyeing the water with distaste.

Assuring her grandparents that she would be fine, I took the little girl by the hand, using my quiet voice. My heart broke seeing her eyes brimming with tears. We edged closer, then stepped into the water. Her viselike grip squeezed the blood out of my hand. We climbed down together onto the second step, then the third. Her grip grew, if possible, even tighter.

"Splash me," I suggested. Looking me in the eye to be sure I meant it, she bent down and scooped up a small handful of water, pouring it onto my leg. I splashed her back. Bringing a hand full of water to my face, I blew some bubbles. Motioning to her, I held the water in front of her. Eyes fixed on mine, terrified of what might come next, she just touched her lips to the water's surface. She blew, as though cooling off a blistering hot cup of tea.

"We're going into the water now; I'll hold onto you," I promised. Assuring her I would not let go seemed unnecessary, since she clung to me like a leech. I couldn't have let her go if I'd wanted to.

Through tears and hysterics the words stuttered out of her mouth. "You promise?" I promised, then dropped a bomb. I was going underwater—with her. She thought this was a pretty bad idea, and began protesting—loudly.

Suddenly a childhood memory came to mind. My best friend's sister was standing in front of her mother, waiting to get her hair combed. As her mother combed through her fine, snarled hair, the child's wails reached a crescendo. I stared, transfixed. My friend wanted to go play; she'd witnessed this scene way too many times. I, however, had never observed this amount of energy expended by a mother or daughter to get hair combed. This had never happened at my own house.

The hair-combing ritual winding down, my friend's mother became playful with her younger daughter. Smoothing out one snarl, she stopped combing as her child continuing to wail. Comb poised over her daughter's head, the mother pointed out that she wasn't doing anything to her; she needed to stop crying. The wailing finally stopped. Her mother then said, "Ah, there's another snarl, you'd better start crying," whereupon the child set to howling yet again. As her mother teased out one tangle after the next from her daughter's fine hair, the child turned her tears off and back on like a well-trained actress. This drama promised to continue for a while. Tearing myself away, I left with my friend, yet the scene stayed with me.

My attention drawn back to the present, to the pool I was standing in, I spoke to the child in my arms. "We're going to go under water. When we come up, you're allowed to yell as much as you'd like. Why don't you practice now?" As she bellowed, I congratulated her. "Good job! Now, when I say we're going under, you'll do better if you close your mouth and stop yelling. Otherwise you'll get water in your mouth and it won't feel good." Her eyes grew wide, and she clutched, if possible, even tighter; so much the simpler to get her underwater. "We're going under," I warned. "Better close your mouth," then held her close as we went under the water, her mouth clamped shut. Once back above the surface, I said, "Ok, you can start crying." My suggestion was unnecessary.

Encouraging her to cry, then going back under together, we came up to lots of spluttering and crying. After uncounted trips up and down together, we emerged, and I said, "You can cry now."

This time however, something had changed. Taking a big breath, she looked around in bewilderment and said, "The tears won't come." I looked at her and chuckled, and then we laughed together.

From there she moved to floating on her stomach, and blowing bubbles with abandon. She practiced kicking, discovering that she could move in the water with ease. Her grandparents stood by the side of the pool, smiling from ear to ear.

This reluctant child became my most eager and determined of students, arriving to class first, leaving the water last, playing, and reveling in how the water buoyed her up. From fear, with some hand-holding, and body-clutching, she moved to joy.

I have put these lessons into practice in my own life as it has taken many unexpected turns. Family and friends along the way have made the difference in helping me face many situations that have felt scary. Searching for and finding Easy Walks wherever I am has been another step along the road. Bringing others with me on the journey has increased my joy.

Anxiety about an undertaking does not imply a lack of desire; sometimes the feared activity is what we most need. Reluctance can be a signpost, a clue that there may be something important beyond the fear. Being offered a firm and kind hand for a season is just what some of us need. A dash of imagination doesn't hurt, either.

No Longer Afraid—2011

Glancing through the glass window, she tucked an unruly lock of her dark, shoulder-length hair behind one ear. She leaned inside the office door, her dark eyes scanning the room; her knee-length skirt covered substantial hips.

"Marisol?" she asked, hoping my co-worker was nearby. My eyes darted through the crib sheet on my desk, hoping to fix on a useful phrase. "Marisol não está aqui," I told her—Marisol isn't here. I read with care from my "cheat sheet," the unfamiliar syllables of Portuguese tumbling awkwardly off my tongue. The woman nodded, drew her head back and strode off.

My pulse slowed. I had begun work in 2001 at an agency in Milford, Massachusetts that offered help to young families. A number of our clients were from Portuguese and Spanish-speaking families. Our English as a Second Language (ESL) classes drew many inquiries. Each day I struggled to make myself understood by those whose second (and sometimes third) language would one day be English. Some day, but not the day they walked through our door.

My Portuguese was non-existent, and my only Spanish lessons had been in fourth grade, the highlight of which was the staging of Goldilocks and the Three Bears. In the role of Goldilocks, I was to bellow, upon sighting the three bears, "Tengo mucho miedo!"—I am very afraid! Evidently my performance was quite convincing.

Having had no way to immerse myself in another language, in this job I was plunged into the deep end, finding myself in another culture, each day meeting immigrants who knew no English. My limitations were obvious to them and to me, and frustrating for all of us.

The telephone presented me with a deeper level of discomfort. In person I could convey remarkable amounts of information with hand gestures, shrugging, or shaking my head. My large desk calendar helped clarify dates. Phone calls, however, begat much confusion, voices being our sole means of communication. "Não falo Portuguese"—I don't speak Portuguese—felt like an inadequate response during these stressful encounters.

Marisol suggested I meet her friend Renata, a former elementary school teacher from Brazil. Renata offered Portuguese reading and writing classes to Brazilian children. These were skills parents wanted their children to learn to assure they could communicate with grandparents and other family members who remained in Brazil. They would not learn to read or write their native tongue in American schools. She agreed to add me to her student roster.

The narrow stairs to Renata's apartment led me into an even more intense new world. While her students labored over their Portuguese worksheets, Renata endeavored to teach me the language. She smiled, yet most of what I heard her say was unintelligible. I listened with incomprehension while Renata directed her young charges. They understood what she told them. The strange rhythms and tones of Portuguese conversation washed over me, drawing me into a new experience of language. I tried to remember phrases. The children glanced over at me and grinned.

Renata knew little English; our conversations became comical exercises of jumbled sentence fragments in English and Portuguese. We spent half the time on my studies, the other half on English for Renata. "Dificil," Renata muttered with a discouraged shake of her curls, her brow furrowing as I encouraged her to try simple English phrases. Upon resuming my Portuguese lessons, however, her confidence returned. She often said that I must "práctica, práctica," assuring me that this was the secret to learning another language. Her kindness, sense of fun, and willingness to tell me of her own struggles washed away my fear. I found encounters with those w ho spoke little English to become less stressful as I continued my studies.

One day a young couple stepped hesitantly into my office. Suspecting they were Brazilian, I greeted them. "Tudo bem?"—Everything's fine? "Tudo bem,"—Everything's fine, they agreed, their faces brightening at my welcoming phrase, spoken in Brazilian Portuguese. A torrent of words cascaded over me after these social niceties, and I was soon overwhelmed with language that beyond my comprehension. Hoping to get back in the game, I requested, "Fale devegar, por favor"—please speak slowly. Nodding, they smiled, looked directly at me and enunciated careful, simplified phrases. I grasped enough of what they said to respond appropriately. After they left, I felt startled that I had conversed with this family solely in Portuguese. I had understood them and been (I hoped) understood. With each similar ensuing conversation, more and more pertinent Portuguese phrases came to me with ease.

While I studied with Renata, I also spent time at home listening to Portuguese movies and Spanish "novellas," somewhat akin to American TV soap operas. My comprehension of Spanish increased with this submersion in yet another language similar to Portuguese; however I had fewer occasions to interact with native Spanish speakers.

A young mother from Guatemala smiled as she entered my office. Her short stature and shiny black hair reflected her Central American Indian heritage. We spoke alternately in English and Spanish. She answered my questions about life in Guatemala, her family, and the differences she observed between her native country and the U.S. "I like it here. I don't hear gunfire at night," she confided. "I can also wear my wedding ring. In Guatemala, any jewelry I wore would have been stolen."

One day I said something to her in Spanish and she giggled. "What is it?" I asked her.

"You are speaking Spanish with a Portuguese accent." We laughed together at my confusion as I straddled the different languages that bubbled through my office.

With the loss of agency funding, my job ended, and with this loss, regular reasons to interact with immigrants in the area were removed as well. I no longer "práctica, práctica" and my Portuguese and Spanish skills have declined markedly.

Several years after I had last spent time working with local immigrants, we visited my dad in Florida, and went to a nearby bird sanctuary. As we strolled through the aviary enjoying the tropical birds moving about unencumbered in the large enclosure, a young dark-haired girl being pushed in a wheelchair came toward us. Her hands clasped over her head, she cried out in Spanish, "Miedo! Miedo!"—I'm afraid!

The birds were beautiful yet all had been injured, unable to fly; her fears were unfounded. I searched my memory for simple words that would assure the child; the languages I'd worked so hard to acquire had eluded me in the years since I had left the center for families in Milford. I recalled one simple phrase, and spoke directly to the child, (in Spanish) "No peligroso"—they aren't dangerous.

Dropping her hands, she gazed at the birds that surrounded us. She understood. I continued, "Qué lindo,"—how beautiful; I smiled and indicated the colorful birds. She smiled back, then spoke to her mother, pointing at the huge wood stork that had frightened her.

Moving away from the girl and her mother, I thought to myself, "No tengo miedo"—I'm not afraid. No; not so much anymore.

In the four years I spent working in this nearby community I discovered a world that was quite different from my own. I felt such respect for these brave travelers who had had the courage to leave home and all that was familiar to immerse themselves in a country, a language, and a culture so different from their own. My work in those years helped me see that I too had much to give, not in spite of, but because of the difficult experiences I had survived and learned from. What strange, strange grace, indeed.

Acknowledgments/Final words

I would never have started writing seriously if my cousin, Em Turner Chitty, had not challenged me to do it every day. Many of the essays in this book would have been lost if Ben Chitty, a librarian by training, had not cataloged and preserved my writing. After an unfortunate computer accident, he was able to return to me many of the stories included here. Thank God for the sensibility of librarians everywhere.

Thanks to Bri Obed, a writer for Gordon College's alumni magazine, for the title of this book. She interviewed me and headlined her profile "A Liturgy of Easy Walks." She gave me her blessing to use this as the title of my book.

Mary Glen Chitty helped organize chapters, sort out themes and provided a final read-through. Beth Nelson has been a one-person cheering squad throughout the process of writing this book. Phil and Rob Kuhl have been there when I needed them most. Caleb Rae and Anna Rogers gave me a reason to keep going and continue to cheer me on. My grandchildren, every one of you! make my life brighter every day. Thank you, Aunt Betty, for teaching me to swim and for always loving me.

Rob Fitzpatrick and Devin Hunt invited me to test out the "Helpthisbook.com" tool for use by my beta readers. Our "Write Useful Books" accountability groups have kept me focused throughout the writing of this book.

Thanks to each beta reader: Amy Bartelloni, Reverend Merritt Schatz, Reverend Christine Keddy, Robert Perry, Julia Ramsey, Libby Atwater, Pat McNees and others. If I have missed anyone, please forgive me and know your work through the helpthisbook.com beta reading tool made a difference.

My Bellingham, Massachusetts writing group offered encouragement as I read portions of this book during the past year or so. You are talented writers in your own right.

Sue Stephenson performed magic transforming my photograph into the cover design of this book. You made this a book cover that I love. Thank you.

Francie King provided invaluable copyediting. Additions to the manuscript after her work was completed have surely introduced mistakes, which are my own.

Chris Richardson and Rose White: for all you did while you were here. I think of you every day. Thanks to Ellen Chagnon, Sue Richardson, Barbara Monaghan, Carolle Lawson, and Jennifer Powell, for friendship, encouragement, and being there. To everyone who has taken a walk with me, I am grateful for your friendship, support, and encouragement through the years. Thanks to Liz Myska, who opened my eyes to the world of visual impairment.

Bob Golder, for the "Marjorie" Dances, and for all the dances we have enjoyed together over the years. Jay Borden, for working with Jon to build a tandem bike I could ride.

My husband Jon helped me discover what Easy Walks are all about and is my favorite dance partner. He encouraged me to adopt hiking poles, a tool that has increased my independence. Thanks for getting me through the craziness of computer stuff, and always being there, no matter what.

I was hoping the stories within this book would have the final say, while some thought I should provide an additional word. I hope these acknowledgements offer a picture of how extensive a community it can take to help a person find her way.

We've come to the end for now. I look forward to continuing the conversation wherever it takes us. Readers, your feedback is welcome—Marjorie@marjorieturner.com is where to find me. Reviews are much appreciated. Thanks for reading, and Happy Trails!

Made in United States
North Haven, CT
16 April 2022

18325656R00108